Rescuing Our Youth from the Porn Trap

It is time to acknowledge that almost all of our young men, and many of our young women, have been exposed to pornography.

A large number of them have become fixated on it. There are many voices emphasizing avoidance, but few are actually rescuing those trapped in this most damaging and addictive activity.

This guidebook is designed to educate and equip parents to better understand the pornography pandemic, provide protection and, if needed, provide tools for healing.

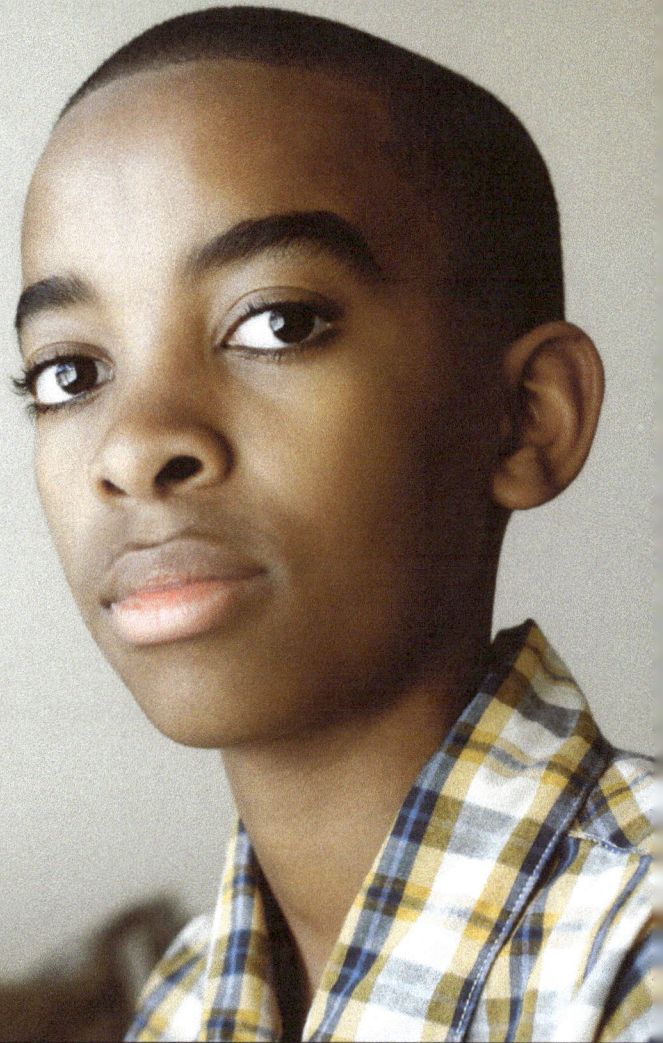

RECLAIM +

GOD'S PLAN FOR **Sexual Health**

A PARENT PRIMER

RECLAIM SEXUAL HEALTH RESOURCE

PRODUCED BY

ELIZABETH MINISTRY INTERNATIONAL

Through *Reclaim God's Plan for Sexual Health* programs and resources, *Elizabeth Ministry International (EMI)* brings hope, help and healing to those caught in the trap of pornography and other unhealthy sexual behaviors. Along with an online recovery program, EMI offers help for teens, parents, spouses, clergy, and teachers.

For information regarding the full range of
RECLAIM GOD'S PLAN FOR SEXUAL HEALTH
books, audio CDs, training DVDs, online recovery program,
healing tools, faith resources, keynotes, trainings, workshops
and retreats, please visit our website at:
www.reclaimsexualhealth.com
or call 920-766-9380

"RECLAiM addresses one of the most serious attacks being waged on the family today! I have personally asked Elizabeth Ministry International to take on this challenge and ask you to do whatever you can to support this vitally important ministry of hope."

The Most Reverend David L. Ricken
Diocese of Green Bay

© 2014 Elizabeth Ministry International - RECLAIM Sexual Health Division
120 W. 8th Street Kaukauna, WI 54130
www.reclaimsexualhealth.com
Phone: 920-766-9380

Primary Authors: Bruce Hannemann, M.A., Jeannie Hannemann, M.A., Mark Kastleman

Contributing Authors: Kristin Bird, M.A., Carol Quist, M.Th, Paul Quist, MDiv, STL, Chris Sperling, MA, LMFT

Editing: Abbi Garavet, Julie Kresal, Don Warden, M.A., Christine Wert, M.A.

Cover Design and Internal Illustrations: Mary Smits

We wish to express gratitude to the many therapists, scientists, theologians, clergy, teachers, youth ministers, teens and parents who have shared their wisdom and experience with us to make this book possible. We especially want to acknowledge the contributions of the RECLAiM Team of professionals.

This book does not constitute medical or psychological advice for treating addiction. It is meant for educational purposes only.

Rescuing Our Youth from the Porn Trap - Parent Primer, 2nd Edition   ISBN: 978-0-9855828-6-9

www.facebook.com/RECLAiMSH   @RECLAiMSH

TABLE OF CONTENTS

This resource and all the works of RECLAiM have been consecrated to Our Lady of Good Help by Bishop Ricken.

OUR LADY OF GOOD HELP
TEACH US TO EDUCATE CHILDREN
IN THIS WILD COUNTRY

The Shrine of Our Lady of Good Help is the only approved apparition site in the United States. The Blessed Mother appeared to Adele Brise in 1859. She told her to "Gather the children in this wild country and teach them what they should know for salvation." Truly we need to follow her words in today's wild, sexualized society.

A Message From A Therapist

"Consider that the average age most children are exposed to pornography is 6th grade. Now consider that 11 years old is the time when most children truly become aware of their sexuality for the first time. It is no wonder that pornography so easily becomes a lifelong habit for some. Pornography teaches us that we are controlled, dominated, and completely defined by our sexuality and our sexual experiences. Learning this false lesson leads many to chase from sexual experience to sexual experience throughout their lives without ever fully living as our loving God intends. We can never fully live if we are only existing for one part of our being. The powerful pornographic images that misinform consciences and lie about what sex is REALLY about at this critical age, skew our children's understanding of who they have been created to be, of the nature of marriage, and of the beauty of their sexuality.

Saint John Paul II, in his "Letter to Families" told us that parents are to be the first teachers of their children.* Included in that instruction is the demand that we must not hide from teaching our children about sexuality. They must be taught the true lessons about the appropriateness and beauty of this part of them, and that it is just one part of who they are – not the totality of who God created them to be. We need to teach our children to integrate their sexuality, in the appropriate unitive and procreative manner, into the totality of who God created them to be. The first step in teaching them this lesson is protecting them from learning the false lessons and the lies of pornography in the first place. Second (which must begin before 11 years of age) is teaching them about what a beautiful gift sexuality is within a loving and sacramental marriage, and that delayed gratification is a way to honor this gift. Teaching these truths at this critical age (and beyond) will combat the lies of our pornographic culture and help them appreciate sexuality as entering into creation with God. They will be able to see that the sexual dimension of a sacramental marriage is one way they can image the God in whose likeness they have been created.

If we model these truths in our lives as parents, teach these truths to our children, and do what we can to protect our children from lies that distort these truths, we stand a far better chance of winning the battle against pornography. It is not an easy battle, but we must be prepared to take this battle head on. Our children are worth it.

As a Catholic therapist, I am always looking for quality, faith-based resources to offer my clients. The anonymous, online RECLAiM Recovery Program opens up ongoing, daily help that is just not possible for me to provide in my private practice. It helps keep my clients going, and focused on becoming the people of God they are struggling to be, in the hours they are not in my office. RECLAiM's process helps them learn that it is not inevitable to succumb to their struggles and that, while they may have a propensity towards these behaviors, they can make choices in and around their problematic sexual behavior to keep themselves safe from the destruction that follows. The additional resources available through RECLAiM are also very powerful tools. I pray that those who struggle with pornography, and other problematic sexual behavior, find their way to www.reclaimsexualhealth.com to find hope and healing."

Chris Sperling, MA, LMFT
RECLAiM Team Member
Contributing Author

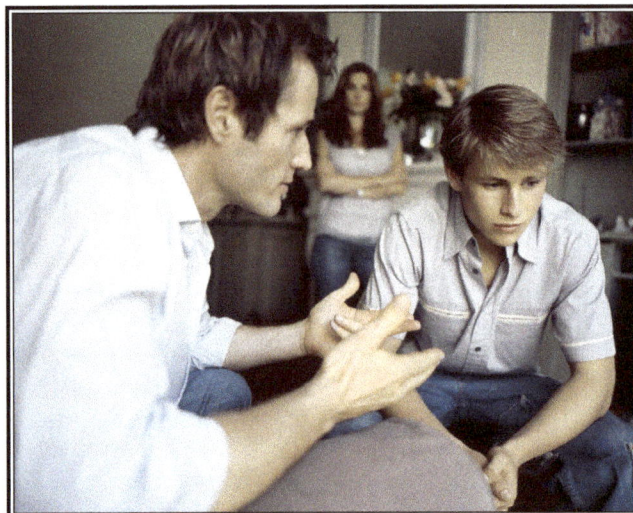

A Message from the Authors

Most parents find it a challenge to talk to their children about sexual issues, especially pornography. However, it is so very important that you talk with your children about the potential for them to see pornography and what to do if it happens. You may not want to discuss this problem, because you want to protect your children's innocence. But the fact is that many children are being bombarded with internet pornography at a very young age. Too often, the child has been exposed to even hard-core internet pornography before a parent would ever think a warning would be needed. Even if you feel your home computer would not be a source, today's children are being shown pornography on their friends' computers, tablets, phones and gaming devices. Despite the Internet's many great features, it engages aggressive tactics to entice your child to view pornography. We have heard too many tragic stories of an innocent child getting caught in the dangers of the web. To learn more about the dangers of the internet and ways to protect your family, go online to www.internetsafety101.org for more information. You can also find more in depth resources at our online store. (www.reclaimsexualhealth.com)

Many children and teens have accidently accessed pornography when they went online to search for a sexual term they heard, but did not understand. If you are the primary educator on these sensitive topics, your child will see you as the source of information instead of the internet. Encourage honest comments or questions. Maintain a consistent dialogue with your child on these topics. Naïve kids are all too often caught in risky online behavior. Having open internet access is unsafe. It is vital to install internet filters and parental control software.

There is a natural shyness about sexual discussions and that is healthy. It is a God-given desire that we be reserved about these sacred and intimate issues. That is why it is important that you, as a parent, be the one to talk about sexuality with your child in a private setting. If you delegate this primary responsibility as parents to teachers or others, your children will usually be taught in a large co-ed group. This desensitizes them and encourages unhealthy sexual behaviors.

Many parents are afraid to talk about pornography dangers because they do not want to put ideas about the degrading images in their heads. Parents can explain the concerns without exploring the images. We teach our children about the dangers of crossing a street, yet we do not go into great detail about the gruesome experience of being run over by a car. We equip them with the action steps of "stop, look and listen before you cross the street." This book is designed to help you instruct your children on the dangers of pornography and provide them with action steps to address the problem. Don't worry, just as you do not need to show or describe to your child an image of a mangled body following a car accident to teach them to carefully cross the street, you do not need to show your child pornography or details of sexuality to discuss the issue.

Along with a warning and instructions on what to do if it happens, we suggest you also address the possibility that your child has already seen pornography. You may be reading this book because you have discovered that has happened. It is vital that you approach your child in a way that does not bring shame or encourage secrecy. Although it may be a knee jerk reaction to scold, blame or reprimand your child, control those urges. Remember your goal is to increase communication in order to protect your child from the dangers of pornography. It is vital that your children feel you are on their side fighting against the evil forces that are trying to cause grave harm. Your children need to know that you are seeking to rescue them, not condemn them.

Not only do you need to teach your children about the dangers of pornography and masturbation, but they must come to understand the beauty of God's plan for sexuality and relationships. Parents and church leaders often explain to children how "bad" pornography is for them, but when children engage in pornography use they experience how "good" it feels. This can be very confusing. Be cautious on how you relate information so that you are not giving the impression that sexuality is bad. You want to teach your children that the pornographers have distorted God's gift of sexuality, and are trying to infiltrate lives with lies. Focus on how unhealthy pornography use is for everyone involved. Invite your child to reclaim God's plan for sexual health. Think of yourself as shining the light of truth on the darkness of pornography's lies.

Bruce Hannemann, M.A., EMI Co-Founder and RECLAiM Co-Director

Jeannie Hannemann, M.A. EMI Co-Founder and RECLAiM Co-Director

Mark Kastleman, RECLAiM Program Advisor

INTRODUCTION

THE PROBLEM

There is a worldwide war being waged between good and evil on the battlefield of the Internet. God's plan for purity is being attacked with the proliferation of pornography literally at the fingertips of anyone with Internet access. The assault is attacking us in every area of life: cultural, moral, political, spiritual, relational and biological. Pornography on the World Wide Web is a stealth strike aimed at our homes and families, a danger that is too often ignored. For safety concerns, parents put their children in car seats, insist teens "buckle up", and make them wear helmets when riding their bicycles, but the same parents seldom implement protection from the grave danger lurking in the electronic world that can be found within today's homes.

The souls of our children are at stake. As you learn about the broad scope of pornography infiltration into the lives of our youngsters and teens, you may feel overwhelmed and want to throw your hands up in surrender. That is what the Evil One is trying to get you to do. Do not give up! There is hope for prevention and healing for those who have already been wounded. The Scriptures have clearly told us who will win this war. In the midst of this battle, we need to remember that God's army of angels and saints are there for us. As you take action to become educated, set in place strategies to protect your family, and seek healing for family members who may be suffering because of pornography, you will experience the power of God's grace to guide you in protecting your children's purity.

In his book, *The Brain That Changes Itself*, neurologist, Dr. Norman Doidge, describes the way pornography causes a rewiring of the neural circuits.[1] The brain center that controls impulsiveness becomes supercharged, and the brain center for willpower shrinks. People who have struggled with drug or alcohol addictions, as well as a pornography addiction, report that pornography was the hardest addiction for them to overcome. If your child is viewing pornography, this re-wiring may have already started to cause problems.

Education about the addictive and destructive nature of internet pornography is vital, and is the primary reason for this guide. Proven tools and strategies are also included to assist you in helping a struggling child. It is necessary to approach prevention and recovery with the same diligence the sex and pornography industry has used to invade our homes and our lives. Only then can we, with God's grace, offer hope to our children and win this war.

Perhaps your children do not have a problem with internet pornography. Give Thanks! Then, focus your energies into serious prevention efforts. On the other hand, you may have accidently discovered that your son or daughter has been looking at pornography, or perhaps your child has confessed it to you. Either way, now is the time to rescue your child from the dark world of pornography. In this parent primer, you will be given information to help your child recover and heal. You will also learn ways to help children avoid future exposure and be prepared if it happens.

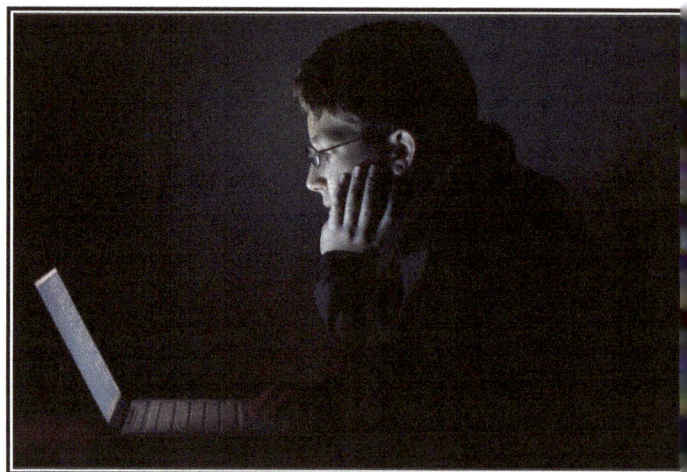

In light of the pervasiveness of pornography use among children and teens, we created this parent primer. It is a basic guide for anyone searching for ways to help children who may be caught up in this evil that is invading our homes. Our purpose is to provide vital information and practical tools parents can use to both protect and heal the purity of their children.

URGENCY FOR RESPONSE

Most parents are unaware of the obscene nature of depraved images and actions that are available on the Internet and free to children of all ages. Access to websites containing sexual and violent images can be gained through not only a computer, but also through cell phones, gaming systems and other electronic devices. If you have Internet at home, pornographers have access to your family.

- Nearly seven in ten (69%) of teens ages 12-17 have a computer.[2] (That doesn't take into account those who view a friend's or relative's computer or computers at local schools and libraries.)

- Nine out of ten children between eight and sixteen with internet access have viewed pornography on the Internet. In most cases, the sex sites were accessed unintentionally when a child, often in the process of doing homework, used a seemingly innocent word to search for information or pictures.[3]

- Cell phones and gaming devices also give access to internet porn and increase the potential for viewing. 93% of teens ages 12-17 go online, as do 93% of young adults ages 18-29.[4]

Between 1998 and 2001, Internet usage among 3-4 year olds jumped from 4.1% to 14.3%; 5-9 year olds experienced a 16.8% to 38.9% increase; and 14-17 year olds experienced a 51.2% to 75.6% hike in internet usage.[5]

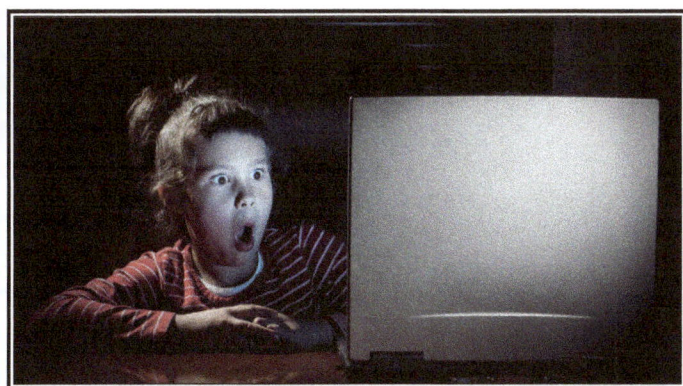

The Internet has brought youngsters nearly unlimited access to information, entertainment, and a variety of ways for social interaction. However, there are the possible risks of sexual solicitation, abuse, harassment and exposure to obscenity in the virtual world that has real world consequences.

As children we have all been afraid of the imaginary "boogey man" hiding under the bed. Today evil truly is trying to enter our homes through the Internet and seeking to harm children. Just like you could turn on the light and discover the "boogey man" was just a jacket laying on the floor, you can remove the fear of online dangers with the Light of Christ. The focus of this guide is how to bring light into this darkness, but before diving into practical tips and methods, you must first be alerted to the extent of the horror that is streaming into your home.

The pornography available on today's Internet is not only naked bodies or couples engaged in intercourse. Any child with internet access can view hard-core pornography that involves sex with animals, children, adolescents, corpses, same sex partners, violence, rape and sodomy. They can also find sexual activities involving inanimate objects, defecation, urination, vomit and other perversions. It has become commonplace to mix sex with gore that includes, violence, mutilation, and even murder.

Exposure to this evil has an impact on children's perceptions of sexuality and on their relationships. Once these unhealthy pleasure connections are in the brain, they can impact many aspects of life.

- *It involves the objectification of people, especially women and creates a mindset of using others.*

- *It creates unrealistic expectations about love, sex and human relationships.*

- *Erectile Dysfunction (ED) due to porn is becoming rapidly common, especially for young men. Habitual masturbation leads to being accustomed to hard friction and some people are then unable to experience much pleasure from normal coitus.[6]*

- *Pornography has become the number one cause of divorce in the United States.[7]*

Avoiding sexual sins will help your child now, in the future, and for all eternity.

PARENT'S ROLE

WHAT TO DO

As a parent, you will need to take the lead in teaching your child(ren) about the dangers of pornography and masturbation. You may also need to teach how to find healing if there has already been active involvement. Because parents often feel this topic can be embarrassing and uncomfortable, it is too often avoided. The dangers are too great and impact too serious to be timid. The following information is provided to promote discussion and offer guidance for you in talking with your child(ren).

To prepare you for this important task, you will need to:

- Increase your awareness of the prevalence and availability of pornography.

- Expand your knowledge of the effects of pornography.

- Intensify prayers for your child(ren).

- Teach your child(ren) faith practices for help, hope and healing.

- Design a plan to safeguard your family and home against pornography.

- Implement healing and recovery tools for members of your family who have become fixated on pornography.

- Inform others of the problem of pornography.

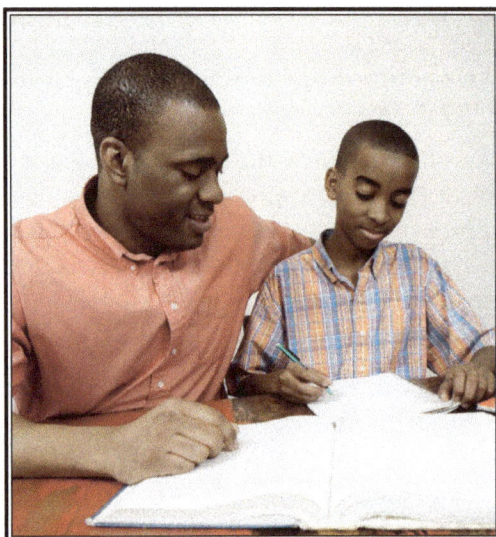

Since every situation is unique, you will need to prayerfully identify the correct response to the dangers of pornography in your home. Use this guide and other resources to obtain information, and then pray to God for the wisdom and courage to respond appropriately.

It is necessary to install filters and accountability software on all your electronic devices, but it is also necessary to guide your children to an awareness of the proper way to respond to pornography, when exposed outside of your home. Teaching your children the correct principles of healthy sexuality and how to establish a moral compass creates an internal monitoring system in your child.

Children and teens are being bombarded with the lies and false promises of those in the pornography industry. The truth is that sexuality is sacred. Do not allow your child to fall victim to the devastation that awaits those who engage in unhealthy sexual activities. Take up the responsibility to teach your child about healthy sexuality and the dangers of pornography.

Parents need to teach their children:

- God has a plan for sexual health.

- There are blessings that come from self-control.

- Pornography and masturbation are against God's plan, and there are serious consequences of unhealthy sexual behaviors.

- God's Divine Mercy, forgiveness and grace are available in the Sacrament of Reconciliation.

- They are loved unconditionally.

It is vital for you to be a role model for your child. A child who sees dad gawking at women, telling sexual jokes or laughing at them, will train his son to objectify others. If mom reads novels and watches TV or movies with inappropriate sexual behaviors, she will teach her children those things are acceptable. Work to heal from your own sexual wounds and struggles in order to model proper behavior.

STEPS TO PROTECT CHILDREN

Vigilant parents can often minimize the opportunities for their children's exposure to pornography, but no attempt will be able to ensure complete protection. Along with your efforts to prevent exposure, be sure to teach your children what to do if they see it.

1. Recognize this is a spiritual battle and pray.

2. Talk to your children about internet dangers, the problem of pornography and what to do if they see it.

3. Use an internet filter on all internet accessible devices. Do not allow the filter to become your security, for none of them are 100 percent effective, and savvy teens can circumvent many filters. Public wi-fi and other's homes may not have filters. Set up safeguards against by-passing filters.

4. Keep all internet accessible devices in communal spaces in the home, never in a child's bedroom. Collect all electronics with screens and disable wi-fi at a set time each night. Password protect enabling or disabling wi-fi.

5. Not all pornography access is through the internet. Sexually provocative material incites curiosity that leads to seeking more stimuli. Do not allow underwear or swimsuit advertisements to be in your home. Monitor the television shows and movies your child watches as many contain pornographic images. Check between mattresses, under the bed or other possible hiding places for magazines or movies that are not appropriate.

6. Monitor use of video game consoles as they often have internet access and movie-playing capability.

7. Check with the parents of your child's friends about steps they have set in place to protect their internet accessible devices. Teach your children to avoid all "screens" in other's homes.

8. Limit sleepovers and campouts. Many young people have been introduced to pornography while at another's home or during group camping trips.

9. Keep your children out of online chat rooms as pedophiles and pornographers often lurk there.

10. Instruct your children about the dangers of social networking sites. They should never share personal information and be very careful about the types of photographs they share. Monitor their activities.

11. Familiarize yourself with family member's cell phones that are capable of receiving and/or taking pictures or video. Check it frequently for pornographic content.

12. Investigate if your child's school library and local community library comply with state and federal laws which require filters on internet access that may be used by children. Take steps to ensure they comply.

13. Review cell phone bills to check for fees which could indicate pornography purchases.

14. If your child uses a smartphone with internet capability, be sure you have had your carrier activate parental control options or install a mobile internet filter.

15. Discuss with your children the dangers of "sexting." (Sexting is sending sexually explicit pictures via text message.) Explain it is illegal along with immoral. Once a picture is sent, it can never be taken off the internet. The sender loses all control over how the image is used or distributed. Monitor, and consider password protecting, the use of all digital cameras, computer cameras, cell phone cameras, etc.

16. Be aware of common sexual text messaging slang and abbreviations:

    - GNOC (get naked on camera)
    - TDTM (talk dirty to me)
    - PRON (porn)
    - NIFOC (naked in front of computer)
    - CD9 (code 9 – parents are around)
    - POS (parent over shoulder)
    - P911 (parent alert)
    - 8 (oral sex)
    - GYPO (get your pants off)
    - IWSN (I want sex now)
    - 121 (private chat initiation)
    - ASL (age, sex, location)
    - DUM (Do you masturbate?)
    - KPC (keeping parents clueless)

WHERE TO BEGIN IF YOUR CHILD HAS A PROBLEM

There are many excellent books, seminars and speakers warning of the dangers of pornography and sex addiction. Unfortunately, most are silent about exactly how to treat these powerful problems. Those that do attempt to offer solutions too often focus on just the spiritual aspects to healing and disregard the important brain training that is also necessary. They may talk about the brain science behind the addictive behavior, but fail to offer exercises that can retrain the brain. Many promote the "just try harder" approach that leads to failure. Some propose that once a person is hooked on pornography, they will forever be in this struggle. This fatalist approach of "once an addict, always an addict" doesn't follow the Scripture accounts of Jesus' healings or the direct reality of God's saving grace.

No trial has come to you but what is human.
God is faithful and will not let you be tried
beyond your strength; but with the trial
*he will also **provide a way out**,*
so that you may be able to bear it.
-1 Corinthians 10:13

Begin with hope in your heart, prayers on your lips, and sleeves rolled up to get to work and help your child experience your support and God's healing!

Keep in mind that engaging in unhealthy and unwanted sexual outlets (porn, masturbation etc.) can create a great deal of shame, despair and self-loathing for your child. Many times he or she may have repeatedly tried and failed to implement the common approach—"Why don't you just stop?" or "You just need to use more willpower!" Many caught in the unwanted sexual-behaviors-trap feel hopeless and think, "Maybe I'm just weak, worthless, a pervert, a freak."

Most struggling individuals, especially children and teenagers, don't understand the specific brain processes that have developed their behaviors over time. Learning there is a logical brain-science explanation for their situation goes a long way in relieving shame and hopelessness.

You will discover that the approach in this parent primer as well as the other RECLAiM resources, combines faith practices with exercises based on cutting edge brain research that are designed to change behaviors. **Keep in mind that there really is a way out!**

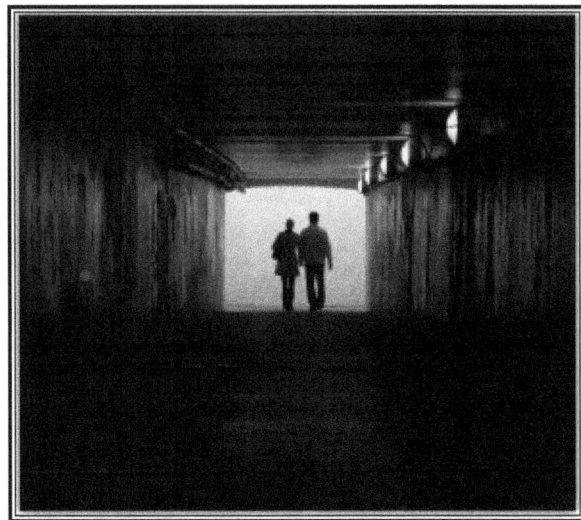

All RECLAiM programs have been created to put a person solidly on the healing path to escape the darkness of sin.

Please keep in mind that this particular resource is very brief and designed to provide some basic knowledge and tools for parents with teens trapped in pornography use. Think of this book as an emergency kit for parents to help you "stop the bleeding" and place your child on the path to healing and breaking free from pornography use and other unhealthy sexual behaviors. For more information regarding our in-depth anonymous, online recovery program, please visit our website at: **www.ReclaimSexualHealth.com**

Note:

Throughout this primer, masculine pronouns such as "he" and "his" have been used when referring to those struggling with pornography. These pronouns are not intended to suggest that this is only a male problem as females are increasingly using and becoming addicted to pornography. Similarly, while pornography addiction can and does impact children at younger and younger ages, this guide often refers to "teens." Many of the practices and activities in this resource can be used by parents seeking to help children of any age or gender.

A PORNOGRAPHY PANDEMIC

A CLOSER LOOK

With the Internet as its carrier, a pornography pandemic is sweeping across America and many parts of the world. It's attacking men, women and children from all walks of life—including people of faith. Unfortunately, like other Christians, many Catholics have fallen prey to this devastating plague.

In a Knights of Columbus article, Pat Trueman, president of Morality in Media, shared this alarming insight:

"In a conversation with a priest in my diocese, I shared my spiritual director's report that every other confession he hears from men involves the sin of pornography. The pastor's response was shocking: 'Oh, it's much worse than that!' Since then, this sad reality has been confirmed by many others: The sin of pornography is overwhelming Catholic men."[8]

In addition to Christian men, there are also increasing numbers of Christian women struggling with pornography. And of course, of grave concern is the number of Christian youth being pulled into this insidious trap. For our young people, pornography is everywhere—on computers, cell phones, video game systems, and cable TV. It can be accessed in many hotels, retail stores, gas stations and most public libraries. Digital porn images are commonly passed around in elementary, junior high, and high school halls, parking lots and locker rooms. The bottom line is that, for most Christian teens, exposure to pornography is a part of their daily lives.

It is estimated that 93 percent of boys and 62 percent of girls are exposed to Internet pornography before the age of 18. And too often, this exposure can lead to various levels of fixation, compulsion or addiction.[9]

This exposure is not limited to the Internet. The average American adolescent will view 14,000 sexual references on TV per year. Turn on the television and you'll be exposed to 6.7 scenes with sexual content every hour.[10]

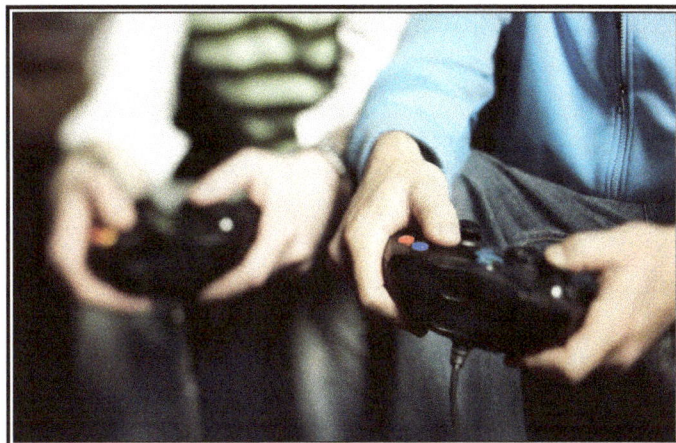

A recent comment from a deeply concerned parent shows the "stealth-like" tactics being used to expose our children:

"I think as parents in this crazy world of extreme media, we have to screen all of the TV shows, movies and video games that our children may play or see. For example, a video game for the computer that is promoted through the public schools for helping kids be more creative and prepared is called MineCraft.™ They even bill it as the ultimate education tool, but I've learned that is has a dark side. My son was over at a cousin's house playing MineCraft.™ They got into a heated discussion about what they were seeing on the screen. On returning home, my son came to us and said, 'No more MineCraft™ for me!' 'Why?' we asked. He replied, 'Oh, because you can buy add-on packages or download them for free and get new levels and skins where you get to choose your own character's skin and many of them are naked women!' We were so proud of him, but for my 12-year-old to be blind-sided by a video game for kids should tell us something—they're trying to implant this stuff into our kids' heads."[11]

All too often parents are simply not aware of the dangers that lurk in video games and other types of technology. This lack of knowledge is leading to a dangerous situation.

"My people are ruined for lack of knowledge!"

Hosea 4:6

HELP FOR PARENTS

PARENTAL PERSPECTIVE

If you've discovered, or even suspect, that your teen, young adult or even younger child is involved with pornography, it's very normal and natural to feel a sea of different emotions that can include feeling:

- as if you've failed as a parent,
- angry at yourself, your child, your spouse, and/or God,
- overwhelmed at the magnitude of the problem,
- confused or disoriented,
- tempted to minimize the problem,
- betrayal,
- sorrow,
- confrontational and lashing out at your child or others,
- deep disappointment and embarrassment,
- helpless and hopeless.

Please know that you are not alone in this roller coaster of emotions! Parents all over the world are facing the same kinds of challenges, including teachers, professional counselors, clergy, and even those who work in the field of pornography addiction recovery. However, while it may be comforting to realize that these emotions are normal and that your family is not alone, this realization doesn't solve the problem.

As a loving, caring parent, how do you help a teen caught in the pornography trap? In this resource, you will find some of the basic knowledge, principles and tools you need to help your teen start down the path to healing and freedom. Remember that additional support and resources are available on our website. Also keep in mind that many of the principles and tools you will learn in this concise resource not only work for healing, but also are extremely effective in helping to protect children and teens from falling into the devastation of pornography compulsion or addiction.

It is important that you take the time to process your emotions, better understand your teen's struggles, gain hope, and provide a clear vision for the healing path that lies ahead.

This process has been extremely helpful for the parents of struggling teens across the world, but, like so many things, you will get out what you put into it. Please set aside the necessary time and energy to carefully consider and complete each exercise in this guidebook. By taking a little time each day, you should be able to complete all of the exercises within a week or so. However, there is no time limit. The key to success is to take the time you need to ponder and internalize the information as opposed to simply getting through it. Turn to God in prayer as you do these exercises. Keep in mind that God's grace is there for both you and your child.

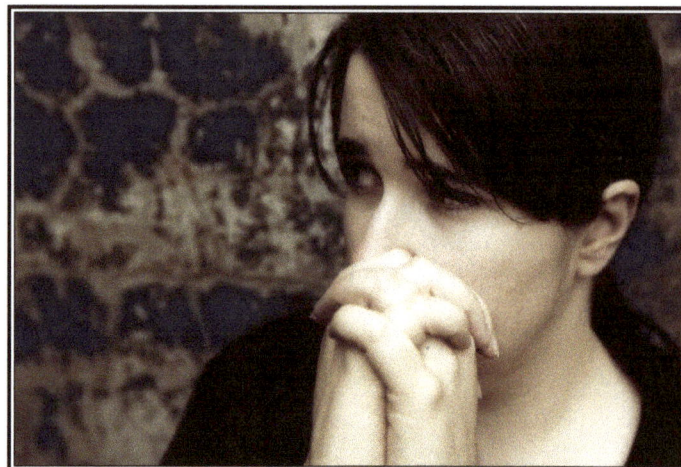

IMPORTANT EXERCISE INFORMATION:

For all of the exercises in this program, you will want to use your own personal and private notebook. You can do this with a paper notebook or journal, which you should keep in a secure location, or on your computer in a password-protected document. What you write is "for your eyes only" unless you feel inspired to share certain entries with your spouse, child, or counselor. Taking this approach will allow you to be completely open and honest while feeling confident that no one, especially your struggling teen, will see your writings unless you choose to share them.

PARENT EXERCISES

Exercise #1: Identify Your Feelings

As you reflect on your discovery of your teen's involvement with pornography, write down a description of each of the feelings that are running through your mind and heart. Consider the list of potential emotions from the previous page as a starting point. For example: "I feel a lot of anger toward my son." "I'm deeply embarrassed that someone in my family would be involved with this stuff." *(Complete this exercise in your private journal.)*

Exercise #2: Identify Your Underlying Beliefs

One at a time, take each feeling that you identified in Exercise #1, and try to identify the underlying beliefs that are causing the feeling. For example, "I feel a lot of anger and disappointment toward my son. I think this is from a belief that he has gone against everything I tried to teach him. Maybe he's not the good kid I thought he was." *(Complete this exercise in your private journal.)*

YOUR CHILD IS A VICTIM

As a parent, one of the first things you may be wondering is, "How could my teenager be involved with this stuff? I thought he was a good kid. What's wrong with him?" Initially, you may feel disappointed or angry, and have a strong desire to confront your teen and express these emotions. It's very normal for a parent to have these feelings, but how you handle them will set the tone for your future relationship with your teen. Impulsively reacting out of anger can have a devastating effect on your teenager's future, including his path toward healing from the effects of pornography. A knee-jerk reaction can trigger shame and drive your teen into secrecy when openness and trust are desperately needed.

Think back to when you were a teenager. No teenager is perfect, and you likely made choices that were not always in line with your parents' values or what you knew was right. Try to remember how you felt when your parents or other adults harshly judged you or put strict punishments on you. This kind of approach can easily ignite the fire of rebellion and shame. Please try to realize that your teenager is not the problem—

pornography is the problem. If you can successfully separate your teen from the pornography, you will start to see more clearly how you can help. Try to see your son or daughter through the loving, and compassionate eyes of Jesus. While you are talking with your teen, set aside your feelings of fear, anger and judgment. This will help your teen feel more comfortable sharing the details of struggles and be more open to receiving your help and support. You can express your pent-up feelings through journaling, in prayer, or confidentially with a trusted friend or church leader.

A teenager who has fallen into the pornography trap is not evil, bad, a loser or a lost cause. In fact, decades of working with thousands of young people has shown that the typical teen falling prey to this trap is highly **intelligent, tenderhearted and spiritually inclined**. These are impressive qualities of religious kids! They are the type Satan is targeting. Remember, more than 90% of kids ages 12 to 17 have been exposed to hard-core pornography, and once they've been exposed, many keep coming back.

Along with their obvious Internet sites, the porn industry also targets our children through online games, YouTube, music videos, cable TV, advertisements, email spam campaigns, website pop-ups, cell phones, merchandise and so much more. They're bombarding our children from all sides. They do this for the same reason the tobacco industry targeted teens years ago. If they can get a child hooked young, they potentially have a client for life. The bottom line is that pornographers are predators who have created a completely unfair and one-sided playing field. Your innocent, struggling teen has fallen victim to insidious tactics and endless assault.

Exercise #3: See Your Teen Through the Eyes of Christ

Take a moment and imagine your teenager with a high fever and body-aches. In this situation, what would be more effective? Your role as disciplinarian or healing physician. To see your child as a disobedient sinner or a suffering patient? Now take a moment and think about the love, compassion and mercy of Jesus. What does Jesus think of your teenager? How does He see him or her? *(Complete this exercise in your private journal.)*

MORE THAN JUST A MORAL ISSUE

THE BRAIN SCIENCE OF PORNOGRAPHY COMPULSION AND ADDICTION

A critical factor in helping you as a parent assist your struggling child is gaining a knowledge and understanding of how compulsive use of pornography is more than a moral issue – it's also a matter of brain science. There are four key insights into your teen's brain that can help you on the path to healing:

• Realize that pornography can create a brain chemical drug addiction.

• Understand how easily the brain progresses from novelty and curiosity to a dependency.

• Recognize how mismatched images, genres and emotions greatly intensify the brain's release of several neurochemicals.

• Develop an understanding of how easily the "neuroplastic" brain forms habits and holds onto them, meaning the ability to change dominant habits is built into the very structure of your teen's brain. Understanding the moldable and changeable nature of the brain will help you see both how the pornography addiction develops, and how God has already given your teen what is needed to break free from pornography or any other unhealthy sexual habits that may have developed over time.

PORNOGRAPHY IS A DRUG

Pornography is perhaps the most mis-understood and underestimated drug in the history of the world. This drug is not injected or ingested. It enters the brain, through the eyes and ears, in a very powerful and real way. Referring to pornography as a drug is not metaphorical. Internet pornography triggers such a radical flood of neurochemicals in the brain, that it has been compared to cocaine.

Now, at the simple click of a button or tap of a screen, people of any age can instantly access unlimited pornographic images from around the world—images that trigger a response in the human brain similar to street drug use. Teens can instantly access this drug from virtually anywhere; it's often completely free of charge, and they can easily keep their use anonymous and secret.

We live in one of the most pressure-filled, stressed-out and fear-laden societies in history. Teenagers have never faced a more challenging time than they do today. Every day, millions of teens are turning to pornography for self-medication and escape from the stress and pressures of life. It has become a culturally acceptable stress release habit.

How can visual images be that powerful? The answer lies in the fact that pornography mimics and counterfeits one of the most powerful forces in humans: sexual intimacy.

One of the most extreme and intense releases of neurochemicals in the brain occurs during sexual activity. The release of these chemicals can be understood using the analogy of an hourglass shaped funnel. The hourglass is wide at the top and slowly narrowing down to a very small passageway in the center and then back to a wide opening at the bottom.

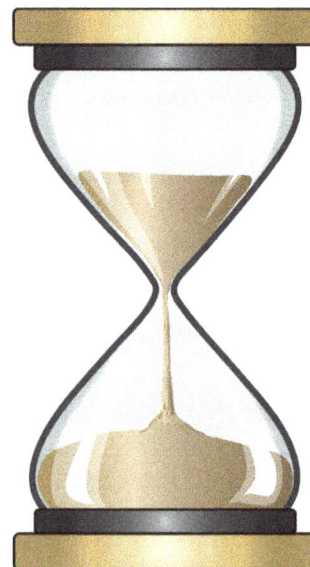

THE FUNNEL EXPERIENCE

As we move through our daily lives, our brain functions at the top of the funnel; it usually has a wide perspective taking in all of the people and things around us. When an individual feels sexually aroused and considers pursuing that urge, the brain immediately starts to release a tidal wave of internal chemicals that narrows its focus; it begins to move it down the funnel. These neurochemicals cause the brain to block out all distractions and focus full attention on the sexual process. The farther down the funnel the brain travels, the more narrowly focused thinking and attention become. Until ultimately, the brain's entire function is focused on trying to get to the very narrowest part of the funnel. This is where sexual climax takes place—causing the brain to release one final wave of chemicals. After the orgasm, the neurochemicals fade, the brain returns to its wide perspective and the full impact of the experience is realized.

Let's look at this "funnel" from two opposite vantage points—first, viewed through the *"Funnel of Love,"* which is God's design for healthy marital intimacy, and second, viewed through the *"Funnel of Lust,"* which takes place during pornography use and other non-spousal sexual experiences. Tracking the function of some of the neurochemicals released during the brain's trip through the funnel experience demonstrates God's grand design for sex and how it can go horribly wrong when not experienced in the right context.

The "pharmacy in our minds" produces many chemicals that interact with this process. Although similar, there are some differences based on the setting.

Neurochemical #1: Dopamine

In the brain, Dopamine has the following effects:

- Narrowly focuses attention and energy;
- Causes us to ignore negatives;
- Triggers feelings of ecstasy and arousal; and
- Creates a powerful dependency.

Dopamine In The *Funnel of Love*

In a healthy marriage relationship this is a wonderful chemical because it causes husband and wife to focus narrowly on each other and to ignore the negatives. (This can be a great benefit to both spouses!) Dopamine also creates a healthy dependency between husband and wife.

Dopamine In the *Funnel of Lust*

The release of this powerful chemical in the *Funnel of Lust* is very similar to the *Funnel of Love*, but the outcome is radically different. Elevated levels of dopamine in the brain produce extremely focused attention as well as unwavering motivation and goal-directed behaviors. This causes the viewer to focus intensely on the pornographic

FUNNEL OF L**O**VE

Sexual arousal with spouse . . .

Stresses, worries and distractions, fade . . .

Intercourse with spouse . . .

Feelings of intimacy, love, and closeness increase . . .

Strong sense of love and unity, with contentment . . .

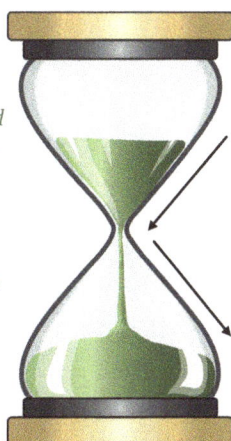

FUNNEL OF L**U**ST

Sexual arousal with porn . . .

Values, willpower, guilt, anxiety fade . . .

Masturbation with self . . .

Feelings of shame, and frustration increase . . .

Strong sense of isolation and anxiety with craving . . .

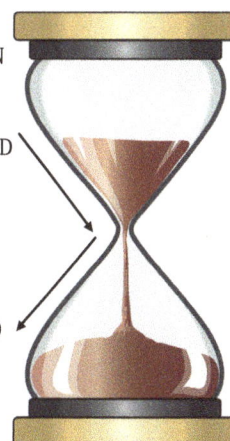

NORMAL DAILY PERSPECTIVE . . . TAKING IT ALL IN

NARROWING FOCUS - LEAVING THE WORLD BEHIND

CLIMAX

RETURNING TO THE BROAD VIEW OF THE WORLD

FULL IMPACT OF THE SEXUAL EXPERIENCE

images at the exclusion of everything else around him. He sees only attractive bodies, only the *perceived positives,* while shutting out all other truth and reality, including thoughts of God, family, beliefs or future goals. All thoughts of negative consequences are blocked out. Dopamine also creates a powerful chemical dependency linked to the images and self (rather than to a spouse).

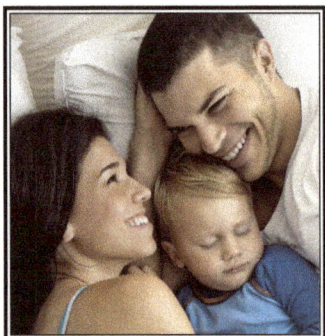

Neurochemical #2: Norepinephrine

In the brain, Norepinephrine has the following effects:

- Generates exhilaration and increased energy through a shot of adrenaline; increases memory capacity; and
- "Sears" the experience in the brain.

Norepinephrine In the *Funnel of Love*

In healthy marital intimacy, norepinephrine brings feelings of exhilaration and increased energy. Each spouse can remember the smallest details of their beloved's features, actions, and cherished moments together. The special and sacred intimacy shared is locked in the memory and can be a strength and a buoy during life's trials.

Norepinephrine In the *Funnel of Lust*

Because of the adrenaline norepinephrine generates, the porn viewer gets a "rush" not unlike that felt while participating in a competitive sporting event or during a thrilling amusement park ride. When viewing pornography, the release of norepinephrine causes the brain to remember every image. This explains why porn addicts can recall the images with vivid clarity years, or even decades, later. Unfortunately, when an individual attempts to overcome pornography use, these images can suddenly "pop-up" in the mind for no apparent reason and result in a constant, frustrating battle to try and keep them out.

Neurochemical #3: Oxytocin

In the brain, Oxytocin has the following effects:

- Emotionally and chemically bonds the two individuals together. When first holding their newborn child, a release of oxytocin bonds a mother and father to their tiny baby.
- This "bonding chemical" is also released when people hold hands, embrace, kiss or even engage in an intimate conversation.

Oxytocin In the *Funnel of Love*

During sexual intimacy within a marriage, a tidal wave of oxytocin is released at climax, forging a powerful bond between husband and wife and producing a feeling of oneness, closeness and attachment. This bond is as strong as the bond a mother and father have with their newborn child.

Oxytocin In the *Funnel of Lust*

When pornography viewing is coupled with self-stimulation and masturbation, oxytocin is released in the brain and body. However, research suggests that the amount of oxytocin released is dramatically less than what is experienced in a healthy marriage relationship. Professionals in the therapy community often report that many teenagers use pornography when they're feeling lonely, disconnected, emotionally needy, and craving real human intimacy. Because the pornography experience is all fantasy, with no real human connection or sharing, the oxytocin release is grossly insufficient and leaves them feeling even more empty, lonely and wanting than before. Unfortunately, this only pushes many to return to the *Funnel of Lust* and pornography, trying to fill the "hole in the soul," which of course, pornography can never accomplish.[12]

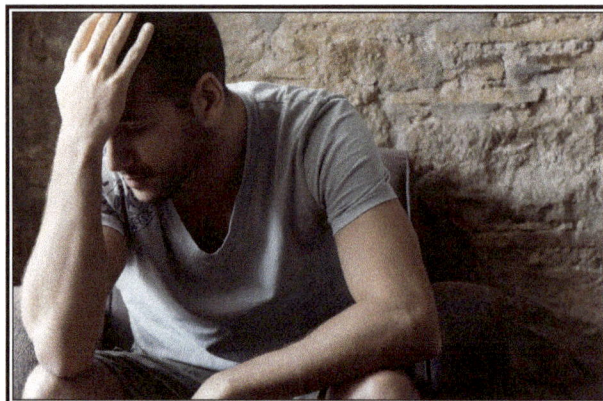

Neurochemical #4: Serotonin

In the brain, Serotonin has the following effects:

- Creates deep feelings of calmness;
- Brings a sense of satisfaction;
- Releases stress;
- Often referred to as the "natural Prozac."

Serotonin In the *Funnel of Love*

Life is filled with trials, challenges and stress. At times, we need a recharging and renewal. When a couple comes together in healthy marital intimacy, the release of serotonin brings deep feelings of calmness and satisfaction with each other and with life. Stress is released, mind and body are refreshed and renewed, and husband and wife emerge better able to meet the demands of daily life.

Serotonin In the *Funnel of Lust*

This natural chemical is released after a masturbation climax, evoking a deep feeling of calmness, satisfaction, and release from stress. Just as those who are depressed may take Prozac to increase their serotonin levels, many individuals turn to porn to self-medicate and escape the stress and pressures of life. This release of serotonin is a big factor in pornography being their "drug of choice."

Neurochemical #5: Vasopressin

Vasopressin is released in the male brain during sexual activity, surging at the moment of ejaculation and climax. It is a bonding and commitment chemical.

Vasopressin In the *Funnel of Love*

Vasopressin strengthens the connection between a man and his wife during the marital embrace. With each successive sexual union and climax, a man becomes increasingly more loyal and protective of his marriage and family. As the commitment strengthens, the man will become more aggressive at defending this relationship, especially against other males seen as a potential threat to that relationship.

Vasopressin In the *Funnel of Lust*

During sexual experiences that occur outside of the marriage bond, such as in the use of pornography and masturbation, a man becomes bonded to himself, the images, fantasies and objects involved, such as the computer. Each illicit sexual experiences reinforces the loyalty to self, to the stimulating circumstances, and to masturbation. A man recedes into a world of denial, isolation, secrecy and narcissism while aggressively defending this unhealthy behavior.

Neurochemical #6: The Hormone Prolactin

During ejaculation, there is a release of brain chemicals, including norepinephrine, serotonin, oxytocin, vasopressin, nitric oxide, and the hormone prolactin. The release of prolactin contributes to the feeling of sexual satisfaction and relaxation.

Prolactin In the *Funnel of Love*

Prolactin levels are naturally higher during sleep and studies show a high link between prolactin and sleep, so it's likely that the hormone's release during orgasm causes a person to feel sleepy. Prolactin decreases the normal levels of sex hormones (estrogen in women and testosterone in men) which leads to the feelings of satiation and delays when a person can have another orgasm.

Prolactin In the *Funnel of Lust*

Men are sleepier after intercourse than after masturbation. Intercourse orgasms release four times more prolactin than masturbatory orgasms. The lower dose of prolactin does not decrease the sex drive. Thus, it is not as satisfying and the search for more sexual release begins quickly, leading to the desire for more masturbation.

A person who engages in compulsive masturbation often will experience problems with concentration and memory. Science shows frequent masturbation causes a drain of the motor nerves, neuromuscular endings, and tissues of acetylcholine and replaces it with too much stress adrenalin. This causes memory loss, lack of concentration, and eye floaters.

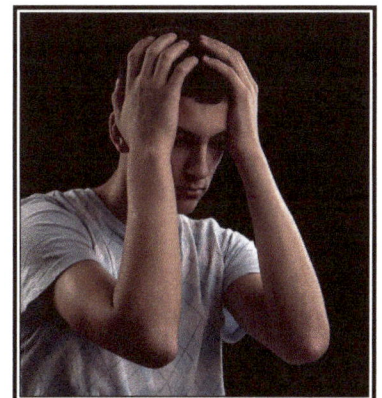

Neurochemical #7: Nitric Oxide

Nitric oxide is a molecule the body produces to help cells communicate with each other by transmitting signals throughout the entire body.

Nitric oxide has been shown to be important in the following cellular activities:

- helps memory and behavior by passing information between nerve cells in the brain
- assists the immune system at fighting off bacteria and defending against tumors
- regulates blood pressure by dilating arteries
- reduces inflammation
- improves sleep quality
- increases your recognition of senses
- increases endurance and strength
- assists in gastric motility

Nitric Oxide In the *Funnel of Love*

Cells that produce Nitric Oxide line arteries. Nitric Oxide allows for adequate blood flow needed for an erection and orgasm. In a normal marital relationship, the frequency of intercourse is usually at a safe level and doesn't cause a drain of Nitric Oxide.

Nitric Oxide In the *Funnel of Lust*

Excessive masturbation causes the liver to release too much nitric oxide into the parasympathetic nervous system. This causes the liver and the parasympathetic nervous system to be overloaded. The result is a deficiency of elements such as Nitric Oxide, which can cause visual problems, such as blurry vision and eye floaters, along with sexual dysfunctions such as impotence, weak erections and premature ejaculation. This is why many young men are now using erectile dysfunction medicines in order to maintain an erection.

NOTE: There are many other physical responses to orgasms. The normal frequency of the marital embrace is healthy. However, excessive masturbation depletes the body's mechanisms beyond what is healthy. Masturbation causes imbalances of the body's nutrients, hormones and other chemicals. This produces a variety of health problems.

GOD-GIVEN POWER AND PURPOSE

This funnel process is so overwhelmingly powerful, the only "safe" place for its expression is within a healthy marriage relationship. Why? Because that's the way God made us! Within marriage, the *Funnel of Love* experience is a wonderful gift that bonds husband and wife together and fortifies every other part of their relationship. Pornography use and masturbation bring someone into the counterfeit *Funnel of Lust*, can quickly become highly addictive, and can literally take over a person's life.

Once pornography plunges the individual into the narrowest section of the *Funnel of Lust*, the brain chemical process is so overwhelming that the individual loses their ability to use logic, reason or think of consequences—free will may even be compromised. When a teen is caught looking at porn, the natural question a parent wants to ask is, "What were you thinking?" The answer is, "They weren't," or to be more precise (from a brain science standpoint), "They couldn't!"

Understanding this basic brain science can help you see why and how your teen could become curious, pulled into, and even trapped by pornography. It explains how pornography use can lead to a brain-chemical dependency similar to the dependency created by street drugs, alcohol and tobacco. Pornography use truly is a chemical, substance abuse.

Exercise #4: The Funnel

Take some time to reflect on this brief overview of the chemical reactions in the brain. Was there anything that surprised you about this basic understanding of "The Funnel" and the similarities between pornography and street drugs? How does this awareness change your perspective of your teen's struggles? *(Complete this exercise in your private journal.)*

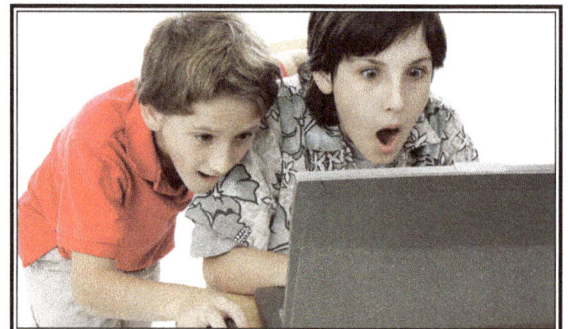

FROM NOVELTY AND CURIOSITY TO DEPENDENCY

NATURAL AND NORMAL

As a parent, it's important to realize that your teen's involvement with pornography probably started out as part of a very normal and natural curiosity. We all have sexual thoughts, urges and desires. In fact, this God-given power to co-create life is manifest in all of us. This includes the power to co-create a human life and to co-create the life of a marriage relationship. Celibate men and women also have this power to co-create, but it is expressed differently through service and spiritual life. Having sexual urges and desires in no way makes a person bad, perverted or evil. **It's what we do with these urges—how we direct this power and this energy, that makes all the difference.**

Pornographers exploit these natural built-in urges, and seek to "hook" our teens over time through a series of stages. The pornographers are the problem, not our teens or their urges!

PROGRESSION OF USE

Many organizations in the recovery movement will offer testing to self identify if a person has reached the point of being a pornography or sex addict. This can give the impression that unless you are addicted to unhealthy sexual behaviors you do not need to be in a recovery program. As Catholics, we have a different approach. ANY amount of pornography use, masturbation or other unhealthy sexual behavior is dangerous. It is necessary to break the chains of any amount of sexual sin. Not everyone who looks at pornography will become addicted to it. Yet, any exposure will cause some toxic ideas about women, sex, marriage and children.

Waiting to do recovery work until the habit has reached the stage of addiction is problematic. It gives a strong hold to this unhealthy behavior in a person's life. It also gives a false sense of the ability to delay purification. Some may respond like St. Augustine prior to his conversion, "Lord, help me to be chaste, but not yet!"

Thus, it is important you do not treat your child's pornography use as acceptable at any stage. Help your child avoid the near occasion of sin. For some, it will be easy to stop the behavior and find healing. Others will struggle and need more support. The following descriptions of the progression of pornography use will help you determine what type of support your child is going to need to purify their passions in order to live a life of genuine, life-giving chastity.

Those involved at Stage 1, 2, 3 can usually break out of the habit of pornography use quite quickly and without long lasting side effects. Those involved in Stage 4, 5, 6, or 7 will need a more focused and intense method of recovery. The sooner the problem is identified, the quicker intervention can occur. As a person moves through the stages, it becomes more difficult to stop. Early intervention is very important.

Stage 1— Curiosity

As children grow up, it's natural for them to be curious about their bodies, the bodies of others, and human sexuality in general. In many cases, experiences with pornography and masturbation start out motivated by simple curiosity. Children can be exposed to these things by accident, through their own efforts, or through friends.

In any case, it's usually natural curiosity that lures them in. If your child's behaviors are at this early stage, with the right education, support and tools, it's often not very difficult for them to break free.

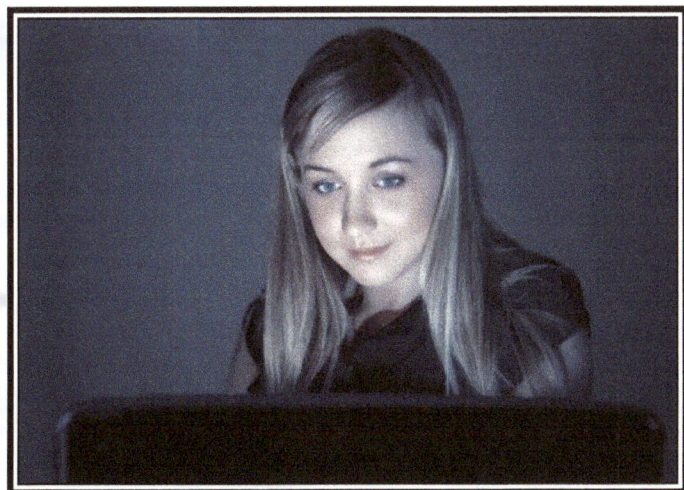

Stage 2 — Experimentation

As children discover pornography they experience an unprecedented stimulation and may begin to experiment with the thrills discovered. Guilt is quickly overcome with the intensity of the excitement. There is a growing overwhelming desire created by physiological changes brought on by the exposure. Too often parents and others consider experimentation a normal part of growing up. Phrases like "boys will be boys" have assumed immoral behavior as normal. This is a dangerous assumption.

Stage 3 — Entertainment

After the initial discovery, many teens start experimenting and then begin using pornography recreationally. They find that it is exciting and arousing. It's a very convenient and powerful way to feel pleasure and to cope with boredom or mental burnout. Pornography viewing and masturbation mimic real sexual intimacy and trigger the brain into releasing powerful neurochemicals producing a "rush" or a "high." Yet, with the right education, support and tools, a person in this stage can quickly make positive progress toward ending this behavior. Without intervention, recreational use is short lived and quickly escalates to a compulsion.

Stage 4—Compulsion

Pornography and masturbation trigger the brain to release the same kinds of neurochemicals commonly experienced with illicit street drugs, alcohol and prescription drugs. What starts out as recreational use can quickly lead to an escalating drug of choice for escape and self-medication. Over time, the teen brain learns that the quickest, easiest, most potent solution for feeling "B.L.H.A.S.T.ed" (Bored or Burned Out; Lonely; Hungry; Angry, Anxious or Afraid; Stressed or Tired) is pornography. For teens in this stage, change takes longer, but with consistent effort, freedom from unwanted behaviors can be achieved.[13]

Stage 5 —Dependency

The move from compulsion to dependency usually happens very quickly. As the dependent behavior escalates, so does shame and self-loathing. Pornography and masturbation now create a "zoning-out" effect that is used as a "self-medication" for anxiety and other uncomfortable feelings. When the shame or other emotions are strong it leads to repetitive escape through more pornography and the vicious addictive cycle is established.

Stage 6 — Addiction

When pleasure is easily and instantly accessible, can be produced on demand, and is experienced repetitively—for example, when internet porn viewing is coupled with masturbation—it can become addictive very rapidly. As a teen repeatedly uses pornography as the primary strategy for pleasure, escape, and coping, the brain begins to believe that this IS the way to deal with the stresses of life. He can get to the point where pornography becomes a central focus in his life. His thoughts become dominated by sexual images, urges and fantasies. Increasing amounts of time, effort and energy are expended on anticipating and preparing to view pornography, actually viewing it, or fighting the urge. Many experts believe that pornography can be a more difficult addiction to break than cocaine.

Stage 7 —Escalation

Once addicted, escalation usually follows. The addicted person becomes desensitized and starts to look for more and more graphic porn. Genres that would have previously disgusted the person, are now exciting. Eventually the person becomes numb to even the most graphic, bizarre and degrading images. This can lead to taking more risks and acting out deviant fantasies in real life. A previously honest person may lie, minimize, manipulate, and avoid the truth of the escalation of addiction.

The teen brain can begin to interpret pornography and masturbation as a "need" just like food or sleep. Over time, the brain becomes dependent on the chemical release that pornography offers. These teens find themselves going back again and again, despite the negative consequences. The stressed out brain is constantly seeking relief and is convinced that it must have pornography to survive—the brain comes to depend on that neurochemical rush just to be able to function in life. Teens at this level of addiction may try to stop, but they can't because they've developed a chemical dependency similar to drug and alcohol addictions. Even those who frequent the Sacrament of Reconciliation and attend Mass regularly may begin to feel that they are such a lost cause that not even God can help them.

If your teen's behavior has progressed to this point, don't give up hope—healing for the brain is possible. Full-on compulsion or addiction takes the greatest amount of time and effort to overcome. Strong boundaries, intensive intervention, and graces from the sacraments are needed—but healing absolutely can be achieved! You may need assistance from a therapist to address underlying or residual issues.

Special Note About "ADHD and Addiction"

According to an article in "*Archives of Pediatrics & Adolescent Medicine*," adolescents with psychiatric symptoms such as attention-deficit/hyperactivity disorder (ADHD), social phobia, hostility and depression may be more likely to develop an internet addiction. If your child suffers with any of these issues, this could help explain some of the reasons behind his or her struggle with internet pornography.[14]

Pornography viewing links emotions and feelings that don't belong together—feelings that don't make sense and aren't compatible: sexual arousal mixed with shock, fear and anger; sexual climax combined with guilt, shame, frustration and hopelessness. This mismatching is the same technique advertisers use to trigger powerful emotional responses in consumers. Pornographers, the masters of this technique, will mix nudity and sexual images with sports, cool cars, beer, food, music, dancing, social popularity, and many other things that are important to teens. But they don't stop there.

Pornographers also link nudity and sex with images of aggression, submission, violence, incest, rape, torture, bestiality, murder and every other form of hard-core imagery they can conjure up. They know the taboo or forbidden induce feelings of shock, fear, disgust, shame and many other negative emotions and that these emotions can trigger a neurochemical tidal wave that is more intense and powerful than the traditional porn images of simple nudity.

This tidal wave of conflicting and confusing images and messages washes over the teen's brain. He experiences feelings of shock, arousal, anger, excitement, guilt, lust, shame, attraction, fear of getting caught, frustration at having "given in" again, and a clutter of other confusing and conflicting messages. These emotions and feelings are directly contrary to the way God designed us to feel during sexual intimacy in marriage, giving rise to conflict and confusion in the brain and triggering the release of an even greater flood of neurochemicals.

Experts have referred to the internet porn experience as a complete and total overload. The human system is not designed to deal with this overwhelming level of conflicting stimulation. We have no natural, built-in coping mechanism for it. (It's challenging enough just dealing with normal sexual temptations!) This is why many therapists refer to internet porn as "visual crack cocaine." In describing its enormous power, Dr. Judith Reisman refers to it as an "erototoxin."[15]

Exercise #5: Your Teen is a Victim

Reflect on the idea of your teen as a victim. How does knowing he is the victim of predatory pornographers make you feel? How does this realization start to change some of the feelings and underlying beliefs you have about your teenager? *(Complete this exercise in your private journal.)*

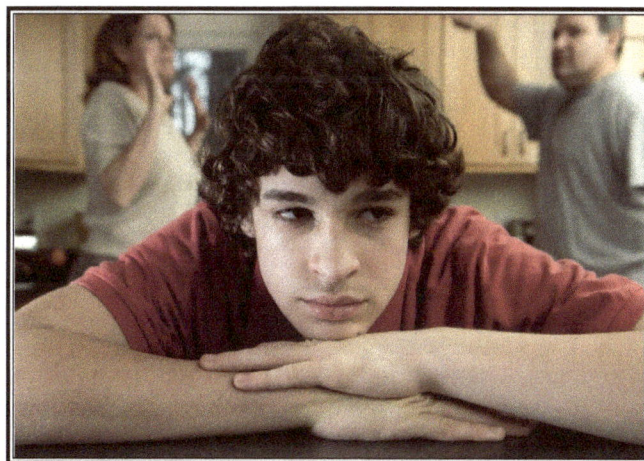

Be sure that, as parents, you unite your teen to fight the evil of pornography. Do not let your child feel his behavior is the source of parental disagreements. Your child must feel the support of both parents in helping to rescue him from the pornography trap.

HOW TO DISCERN IF YOUR CHILD IS INVOLVED WITH PORNOGRAPHY

Because of shame, embarrassment, fear, complacency or denial, teens will often minimize, partially disclose, or keep their pornography use a total secret. Doing so can make addiction more likely because it prevents them from getting the early help and support they need. Unless your teen is completely honest with you, or you catch him in the act, it can be very difficult to discern the exact level of his pornography use. The following are some helpful guidelines.

Stages 1, 2, and 3: The following symptoms could indicate that your teen is moving through Stages One, Two, and Three of pornography use — **Curiosity, Experimentation, and Entertainment.** Keep in mind that these are general guidelines, and do not guarantee that your teen is involved with pornography.

- He becomes quiet, depressed, isolated from friends and family, and discontinues formerly enjoyed pursuits.

- He won't talk about what is bothering him and seems to dislike himself. He is increasingly argumentative, defensive, aggressive and disagreeable.

- His attitudes change: TV programs, movies, pictures and jokes that were formerly inappropriate become acceptable. He begins making comments like: "You have the problem," or "You're such a prude."

- You notice a loss of respect for women and an increased focus on, or obsession with, male and female body parts.

- He begins acting out sexually with self and/or others.

- He stays up late on the computer, locking the door, or quickly switching files or turning off the monitor when someone approaches. He lies about computer use, acting secretive or elusive in connection with the computer.

- Many teens use smart phones, tablets and portable media players like the iPod Touch® to access pornography. If someone approaches, he will quickly turn off the device screen or place it "screen down."

- He may also avoid using these devices when someone is standing behind him.

- When you check the Internet sites he's visited, the history and temporary Internet files have all been erased.

- Your phone costs go up, and strange or unfamiliar numbers appear on the bill.

- He spends a lot of time in internet chat rooms.

Note: In addition to watching for the above signs, an essential component of determining whether or not your teen is involved with pornography is to pray and ask for the Holy Spirit to grant you discernment. God is anxious to grant you this gift. As some parents have experienced "The Holy Spirit can be a beautiful tattle-tale."

Stages 4, 5, 6 and 7: Your teen's involvement with pornography may have progressed beyond curiosity, experimentation, and entertainment into the levels of **Compulsion, Dependency and Addiction.** This may be the case if one or more of the following are present:

- He has tried to stop, but simply can't control the urge

- He can no longer control the amount of time he spends on the Internet or the frequency of the episodes.

- His viewing is accompanied by masturbation, which likely is a way not only to feel pleasure, but also to escape stress, emotional pain or loneliness.

- He finds himself obsessing over and fantasizing about pornographic images when not on the Internet.

- Over time, he begins seeking out images that are progressively more explicit and "hard-core."

Exercise #6: In Which "Stage" is Your Teen?

After reviewing the descriptions of Stages 1-6 and their symptoms, which stage do you believe your teen is in? Write down specific reasons or signs that would lead you to this conclusion. *(Complete this exercise in your private journal.)*

THERE IS GOOD NEWS!

No matter what stage your teen might be in, from simple curiosity to deep addiction, there is GOOD NEWS! Your teen's brain is "neuroplastic" meaning it is moldable and changeable. While consistent pornography use does create a specific circuitry in the brain, that circuitry can shrink and be replaced with healthy behavior circuitry. In addition, your teen's brain will not fully mature until he reaches his mid 20s. Although this can make him more vulnerable to pornography, it can also be an advantage as you strive to help him break free from pornography. While the adult brain remains neuroplastic and changeable throughout life, the teen brain is especially moldable and responds very well to the principles and tools of brain change. The power of habits and neuroplasticity is the hope for your child renewing his mind and breaking free!

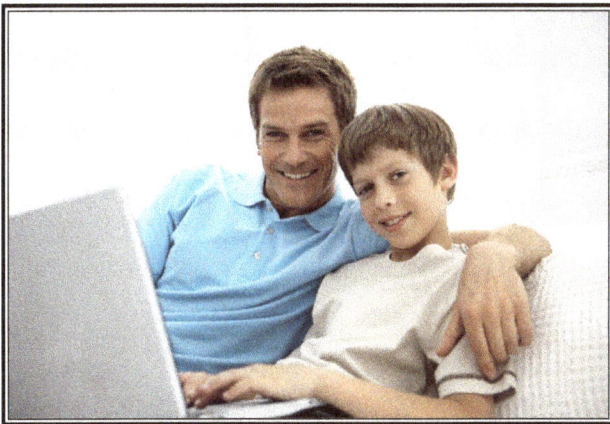

Recovery

Remember that hope and healing are possible at every stage. However, the further down the path of addiction, the more challenging it will be. Keep in mind that once a person has reached the stage of addiction, the behavior has a "hold" on the person and stopping is not the same as just resisting something that is tempting, captivating and alluring. Ceasing addictive behavior involves much more than an act of will. It will take a continuum of care that includes prayer, sacraments, spiritual guidance, education, accountability and a detailed plan. Through the grace of Jesus Christ and a commitment to the hard work of recovery, escape from addiction is possible. Those who have been successful in recovery will have a deepened relationship with our Lord through His healing grace. When someone works on a comprehensive plan of recovery, it is possible to restore sexual health and live in accordance with God's plan.

Spiritual Battle

Always seek the help of the Lord in the process of healing. It is important to cover your family in prayer.

Put on the armor of God so that you may be able to stand firm against the tactics of the devil. For our struggle is not with flesh and blood but with the principalities, with the powers, with the world rulers of this present darkness, with the evil spirits in the heavens. Therefore, put on the armor of God, that you may be able to resist on the evil day and, having done everything, to hold your ground. So stand fast with your loins girded in truth, clothed with righteousness as a breastplate, and your feet shod in readiness for the gospel of peace. In all circumstances, hold faith as a shield, to quench all [the] flaming arrows of the evil one. And take the helmet of salvation and the sword of the Spirit, which is the word of God. Ephesians 6:11-17

Parental Support

The most powerful aspect of recovery for a child who has been caught in the pornographer's trap is parental support. The more time you spend uplifting and encouraging your teen, the more your child will have the strength to continue doing the work of recovery. So often a child feels they are "bad" in your eyes if they have done something wrong. Be sure your child understands you believe he is good, but is caught up in a bad thing.

As parents, you can get support in your efforts through RECLAiM Sexual Health. You can enroll in a free parent support resource that will guide you in ways to assist your son or daughter. (www.reclaimsexualhealth.com)

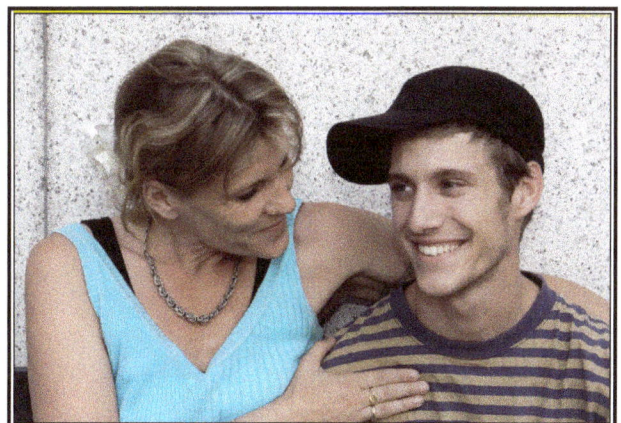

UNDERSTANDING MORE

THIS IS <u>NOT</u> THE PORNOGRAPHY OF DECADES PAST

Some parents have a hard time understanding how pornography can create such a deep and difficult chemical dependency and addiction. One father exclaimed, "Why is my son having such a tough time with this? What's the big deal? I remember Playboy Magazine when I was a teen. It was something you looked at and then you moved on. I don't get why this should be such a major problem."

Today's internet pornography is not the Playboy Magazine images of decades past. The Internet has changed everything. Consider the state of online pornography today:

Novelty and The Brain: The human brain loves novelty, newness, variety and the unusual or out-of-the-ordinary. This is especially true of teenagers—they can stand just about anything but boredom! There are over **42 million** pornographic websites on the Internet (nearly **half a billion** pages of porn images and videos), and many cost nothing to access. This is a practically unending supply of variety to feed the bored teenage brain. Because the brain craves novelty, this variety factor alone hooks many teens.

In addition, in the old days of magazine pornography, there were a limited number of images in a narrow genre. Many people would see the images, and once the initial novelty and excitement wore off, they would become bored and move on. Today, Internet porn makes that boredom impossible. There are hundreds of millions of porn images of every possible variety and dimension—anything and everything can be imagined, even much that many would consider beyond human comprehension. Some believe, "I could never be pulled into that smut!" But with the astronomical variety of images and genres of Internet porn, if a person browses long enough, eventually they will encounter something that "hooks" their curiosity. This is what leads so many to be vulnerable.

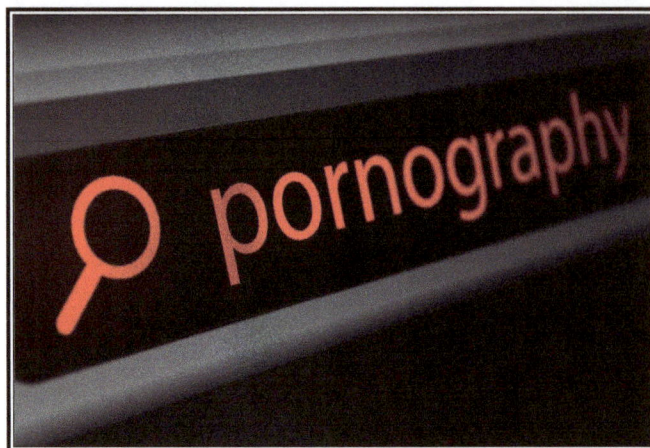

The experience is more than just sexual: There's a lot more going on with today's online pornography than just sexual arousal. Internet porn triggers a vast array of emotions, feelings and memories that have nothing to do with sex. It's these "other" factors that give pornography an enormous power that goes beyond the sexual.

Today's internet pornography is very different from the print forms of it in the past. It offers an endless stream of variety allowing a user to continually seek new sources of dopamine levels. The chemical rush is available 24/7 and much of it is free. Dr. Jeffrey Satinover of Princeton University has said, "It is as though we have devised a form of heroin ... usable in the privacy of one's own home and injected directly to the brain through the eyes."[17]

If a person's brain gets used to being flooded with these chemicals, trying to stop the use of pornography leads to withdrawal symptoms. At this point additional problems in the brain have most likely occurred. The part of the brain (frontal lobe) that helps a person think through circumstances and make good choices gets damaged.[18]

When you discovered your child was using pornography, did you say "What were you thinking?" Well, now you know a possible answer. Your child wasn't thinking! The part of the brain designed to think, reason and apply moral judgments is broken and not working.

WHAT'S HAPPENING?

Pornographers promise healthy pleasure and relief from sexual tension, but what they often deliver is an addiction, tolerance, and an eventual decrease in pleasure.[19]

—*Norman Doidge, MD, The Brain That Changes Itself*

It is important to look at what is happening in the brain of someone who gets hooked on pornography and masturbation. You do not have to be a neurosurgeon to have a basic understanding. Let's start by looking at the "reward pathway and motivation circuit" that is deep inside of the brain. Its job is to reward a person when doing something that promotes life. Two of our major reward responses are related to staying alive (eating) and creating new life (procreation). Rewards for life sustaining activities are accomplished by releasing chemicals in your brain that make a person experience pleasure. Dopamine is one of the powerful reward chemicals that make a person feel good.

Normally, dopamine and other chemicals are what help us feel pleasure and bond to one another. They are the motivation that keeps us coming back to important activities. However, the problem is that this reward pathway can become hijacked by activities that produce the same chemical response, but do not promote life.

For example, cocaine makes a user feel a high that releases these reward chemicals without having to do the work to earn it. Pornography does the very same thing. The surge of chemicals creates new brain pathways that condition the user to repeat the behavior that provided the strong rush of chemical pleasure. The more the person uses pornography, the more those brain pathways get wired into the brain to create an automatic behavior, even if the person does not want to do it.

Eventually, this continual overload of chemicals causes other changes in the brain. For one, the brain builds up a tolerance as it adapts to the higher levels of dopamine that pornography use releases in the brain. In an attempt to protect itself from the overload of dopamine, it shuts down some of its receptors. With fewer receptors to

sort of "catch" the chemicals, the brain thinks less is being released and the person does not get the high level of reward feelings. This is the basis of escalation into more hard core pornography or other extreme activities to get the same excitement. This escalation often includes violence and perversions. That is because it is not just sexual arousal that gets dopamine flowing. The brain also releases it when it sees something novel, shocking, or surprising. That is the reason behind so much of hardcore porn showing images of women being physically harmed.

Healthy sexual relationships gradually develop during courtship, engagement and marriage. The limitations of frequency of intercourse within a marriage keep the levels of chemical release at a healthy level. Internet pornography, on the other hand, provides an unlimited opportunity for hyper-sexual images that continually flood the brain with high levels of dopamine, and other chemicals, as fast as the user can click on a new image.[20]

People who use pornography at ever increasing amounts will eventually discover they do not feel "normal" without the chemical high produced by dopamine. Normal activities, like talking with friends or playing a sport, can no longer make them happy, as they cannot provide a high enough amount of dopamine to make them feel good. At this degree of pornography use a person starts to withdraw from activities that once were enjoyed, feels anxious and focuses only on getting the next rush from more pornography.[21]

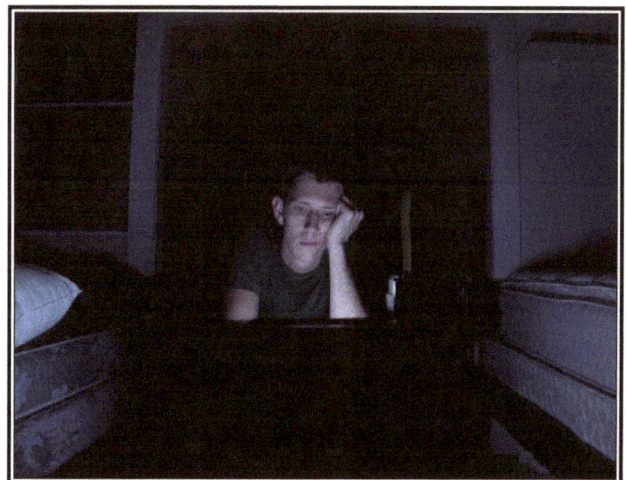

When a person's brain is flooded with dopamine, it is also building a pathway within a protein called "iFosB." This protein helps a person remember to do things that feel good or are important for survival. Dopamine motivates the brain to do something and then rewards it when it has done it. The job of iFosB is to help a person remember to do things and provides a reward for following through with it. iFosB makes pathways in your brain to help you get back to an activity without thinking about it. When this happens for healthy behaviors, it is very efficient and helpful. However, unhealthy behaviors that are rewarded with dopamine also cause the iFosB to establish pathways that lead a person to repeat the bad behavior.[22]

The more a person looks at pornography, the more motivation from dopamine occurs and the more iFosB accumulates. This increases the brain pathways make it easier and easier for repeating the behavior. This can lead to being more and more susceptible to addiction. This process is even more dangerous for teenagers because a teen brain's reward pathway has a response two to four times more powerful than an adult brain. This means teen brains release even higher levels of dopamine and iFosB leaving them even more vulnerable to addiction.[23]

It is important to realize that just because our brain's reward system motivates us to do an activity it may not be good for us. We can see this with desires for sweets. Your brain will produce higher amounts of dopamine if you eat a cookie than it does when you eat a carrot. This reward was based on conditions thousands of years ago when high-calorie foods were hard to find. Years ago when our people came upon a high-calorie food, it was important for survival that they eat it. However, today you can go to the local grocery store and gorge yourself on cookies. This will lead to heart disease, weight gain and other health problems. Today, the drive to eat has become hijacked by junk food in many people's lives.

We can think of pornography as sexual junk food. When a person is viewing pornography, it stimulates the brain to think the person is seeing a possible mating opportunity. The drive to procreate is so strong that the possibility of mating pumps the brain full of dopamine.

Mirror Neurons

If you notice someone yawn, you suddenly feel tired and yawn too. If you watch a sad show, you may begin to cry. If you watch a movie and a scene portrays a surprising and frightening situation, you may feel the need to cover your eyes. This ability to respond to visual stimuli with a keen understanding and take it personally is because of brain cells called mirror neurons. Although it is a movie, you are moved by the images to believe it is really happening.

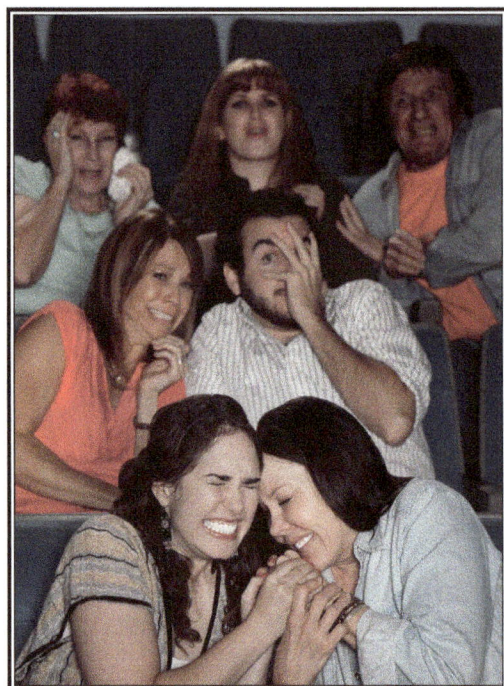

Because of mirror neurons in the brain, viewing pornography does not just cause a person to think about sex. Because of mirror neurons, those watching porn think they are having sex! Pornography works by persuading the brains of people viewing it to believe they are **not watching**, but **doing it**. Fantasy becomes reality to the chemical pharmacy in the brain. Mirror neurons cause those viewing pornography to vicariously experience and learn from what they are watching. This activates sexual arousal causing sexual tension with a desire for a release. The person will act out (usually by masturbating) and set in place hormonal and neurological responses that God created to bind husband and wife. All the chemicals in the brain that were designed to bond spouses are released. Only the bond is with oneself and pornography.

UNDERSTANDING WHAT HAS TO BE DONE TO CHANGE

There is no behavior that cannot be changed, eliminated or integrated into a person's life. The brain has a natural ability for change. The same process of habit formation that got your child caught up in pornography can be used to find freedom from it. Scripture is clear in telling us to be transformed by the renewal of the mind.

Do not conform yourselves to this age but be transformed by the renewal of your mind, that you may discern what is the will of God, what is good and pleasing and perfect.

Romans 12:2

The way to renewal of the mind involves

INTENTION

ATTENTION

PREPARATION

REPETITION

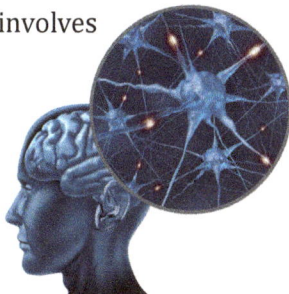

INTENTION: Your teen will need to keep focused on the intention of eliminating the unhealthy sexual behaviors. This will include faith practices that focus on seeking the needed grace to heal.

ATTENTION: Your teen will need to pay attention to the situations and circumstances that can lead to unhealthy sexual behaviors. Emphasis will have to be on "avoiding the occasion of sin." Very few decisions are really neutral. Learning how to discern the path towards perfection is vital.

PREPARATION: In order to make healthy habits, there must be preparation and mental practice so you can make the correct choices.

REPETITION: Repeating an activity over and over is how a habit is formed. Your teen must be careful to make it a repeated habit to choose healthy behavior. Perhaps the following story of the Cherokee Brave explains this best.

Which wolf will you feed?

One evening, an elderly Cherokee Brave told his grandson about a battle that goes on inside people.

He said "my son, the battle is between two 'wolves' inside us all. One is evil. He is anger, envy, jealousy, sorrow, regret, greed, arrogance, self-pity, guilt, resentment, inferiority, lies, false pride, superiority, and ego. The other is good. He is joy, peace, love, hope, serenity, humility, kindness, benevolence, empathy, generosity, truth, compassion and faith."

The grandson though about it for a minute and then asked his grandfather:

"Which wolf wins?"

The old Cherokee simply replied, "The one that you feed."

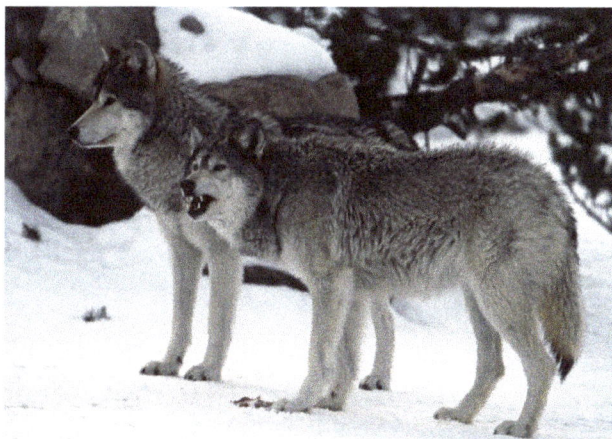

This story helps us reflect on how important are our choices. What a person thinks about and dwells upon will influence behavior.

We each have a choice, we can "Feed the Good Wolf" and it will become a positive habit and show up in our character. We can also choose to "Feed the Bad Wolf" and this will become a negative habit that will turn our whole world upside down while it eats away at our soul.

This is a very important point to teach to your children. The more your teen understands the role of habit formation and neuroplasticity, the better equipped he will be to recover from the damage of viewing pornography.

THE POWER OF HABITS AND NEUROPLASTICITY

REPETITION

The previous pages explained the first three primary characteristics that make internet pornography so highly addictive:

1) The release of neurochemicals can create a dependency similar to street drugs;

2) A vast, ever-changing and never-ending variety of images snare the brain's natural curiosity and hunger for novelty; and

3) A toxic soup of mismatched images, genres and emotions greatly intensifies the brain's release of powerful neurochemicals.

The fourth characteristic is about how repetition causes habit formation. This plays a major role in your teen's continued involvement with pornography.

4) The brain is efficient and will quickly make a behavior that is repeated often into a subconscious action. Repetition leads to the creation of a habit.

Do you remember when your child was little and going through the frustrating process of learning new skills? Tiny fingers awkwardly struggled to tie that first shoelace bow. A nervous hand laboriously scrawled a barely-legible name. When you finally let go, you held your breath and watched anxiously as your wide-eyed child rode a wobbling bicycle down the sidewalk. At first, these simple tasks were excruciatingly difficult and time consuming. But with each repetition the task grew progressively easier until something amazing happened—it became automatic! Through repetition, your child trained his or her brain to turn each task into a habit.

THE POWER OF HABITS

The remarkable power of habit-formation is built-in to the very fabric of the brain and nervous system. Habit formation is the brain's number one priority. Why? Because the brain is dedicated to efficiency. Since the moment your child was born, his brain has focused intensely on being efficient. And the most effective way to be efficient is through the formation of habits. This is what the brain seeks—to focus its energy and attention on mastering a skill and, as quickly as possible, make it automatic—a habit. The brain then moves on to direct its efforts at learning and mastering the next skill. This allows for continual growth and progress.

What must a person do to become really skilled at anything? That's right, "consistent practice." This is the primary method the brain employs to form habits.

While the brain's habit-formation power is a remarkable gift, it can also work directly against a person when attempting to break out of old habits—especially highly advanced habits like addictions. Once the brain expends the time and energy to develop a habit, whether it's good or bad, it doesn't want to give it up.

Imagine what would happen if each time your child tried to walk, speak, tie shoes or engage in any other already-learned skill, he or she had to master it all over again? What if every time you got in your car you had to stop and think, "Now what does this pedal do, and what are these knobs and buttons for?" Without the power of habits, we wouldn't get very far in life.

Once a habit is in place, the brain stamps it with "mission accomplished" and vigilantly guards what it has worked so hard to create. In essence, the brain builds a 20-foot-high, 30,000-volt, razor-wired, super-security fence to protect all its hard-earned habits, boldly displaying the warning sign "KEEP OUT!"

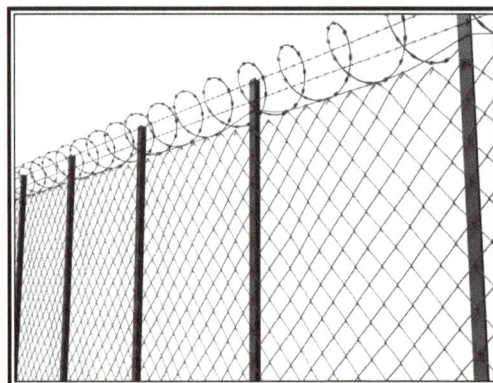

Exercise #7: Repetition and Your Habits

Get a pen and paper and then write your signature five times. Notice that it's the same every time. If you compare it to the signatures of others, you'll find that they're all unique because of individual "repetition" over time.

Now, write your signature with your non-dominant hand. Notice how awkward and difficult it is. Why? Your brain is not "wired" through repetition to do it that way; there's no habit in place.

ADDICTION IS A HABIT ON STEROIDS!

Addiction is the brain's habit formation tendency "on steroids"! Over time, an addiction can be formed if someone has practiced turning to pornography and other sexual behaviors as the most convenient, powerful, and efficient way of instantly escaping boredom, stress, loneliness, and the pressures of life. These outlets have become the brain's automatic, dominant "drug of choice" for escape and self-medication.

Everyone has some behavior they turn to in times of stress. Some outlets are healthy and productive, while others are destructive. Consistently practicing turning to a particular outlet to cope or escape makes that choice automatic, a habit. Over time that habit can evolve into an addiction. A simple definition of addiction is: *the state of being enslaved to a habit at the exclusion and detriment of all other goals and activities. Attempts to stop the habit trigger feelings of withdrawal, discomfort and even trauma.*

With the power of habits in mind, let's take a look at a common situation faced by your struggling teen:

He wants to stop using pornography, but he slips and gives in again. Afterward, under the terrible weight of guilt, regret and self-loathing he declares, "That's it, that's the last time I'll ever do that!" But his brain responds: "Hold on just a minute! Let me get this straight. Just because you're feeling guilty, you expect me to simply abandon this incredibly pleasurable, self-medicating habit that I've worked so hard to build? I don't think so— that wouldn't be efficient!"

The question is, "If through repetition, a powerful habit develops, or even an addiction, can the brain change? Can the circuitry for that habit shrink and be replaced by healthy behavior circuitry?" The answer is YES!

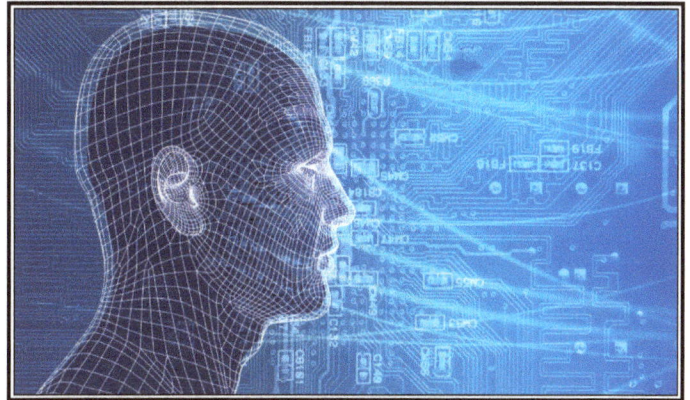

THE BRAIN IS "NEUROPLASTIC"!

The brain is "neuroplastic"; This means that our physical brain circuitry is literally moldable and changeable. In other words, we're not stuck with old negative habits, or addictions. Unwanted behaviors that the brain has "learned" can be "unlearned" and replaced with healthy behaviors.

Whenever we do anything for the first time, the brain puts in place the basic foundation of a habit. Why? Because the brain assumes that we might repeat the action in the future and it wants to make the next time easier, and the time after that easier still. Each time we repeat a behavior, the brain circuitry for that behavior grows stronger, larger and deeper until finally it becomes automatic—a habit.

However, as we choose a behavior less often, the brain circuitry for that behavior begins to weaken—just like a muscle, it begins to atrophy. One of the laws of brain development is "use-it-or-lose-it." Later in this training, you're going to learn a wonderful technique known as "C - IT." You can help your teen use this technique to consistently expand new healthy brain circuitry while shrinking old negative habit circuitry. Your teen will literally learn how to re-shape his own brain circuitry and by doing so, re-shape his life, and reclaim God's plan for sexual health!

UNDERSTANDING THE PARTS OF THE BRAIN

BRAIN ANATOMY AND FUNCTION

It is helpful to learn about brain anatomy and function because it will empower you to understand what is happening within the brain of your child. Knowing about the parts of the brain will enable you to focus attention on the functions of specific regions and promote activities that will ensure healthy maturity for your teen.

This information can help your teen understand some of the things that have happened may not be his fault, but they are his responsibility!

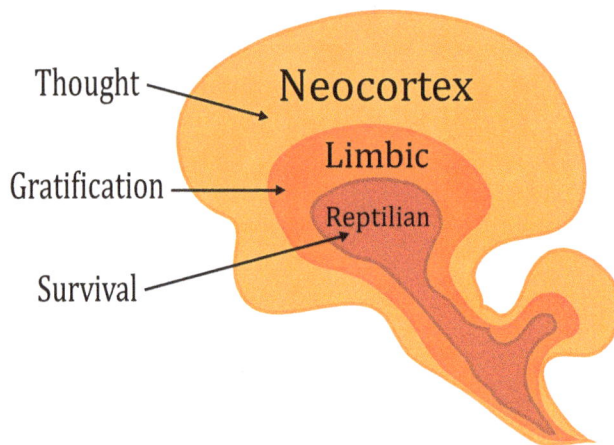

Thought → Neocortex
Limbic
Gratification → Reptilian
Survival →

SURVIVAL – THE BRAINSTEM (REPTILIAN)

The BRAINSTEM, sometimes referred to as the Reptilian Brain, is the portion of the brain at the base of the skill that connects to the body via the spinal column. It is responsible for collecting information from bodily systems for the brain and returning life supporting signals back from the brain to the body to help support life. This includes temperature, heartbeat, blood pressure, eating and drinking, reproduction and survival in crisis or impending threat via the fight, flight or freeze response. Anxiety, fear and other stresses can allow this part of the brain to shut down the other parts of the brain. That is why it is important that your reaction to your child does not produce fear or anxiety as it will keep the thinking part of the brain from functioning properly. This is why Scripture instructs us numerous times not to be afraid. When we encounter fear our cortex shuts down and our limbic takes over and we act like animals - primarily responding with the limbic portion of our brain and without reason or morality.

GRATIFICATION – LIMBIC BRAIN

The LIMBIC BRAIN, the next layer up from the brainstem provides the motivation and emotional drive to follow the basic drives of survival. It contains the reward pathways which provide chemical pleasure rewards primarily dopamine, to ensure that signals from the body and brainstem are acted upon.

This portion of the brain also codes into memory the emotions connected with those signals and responses. It records which actions produced the most rewards so that these actions will be repeated. The memory structures in the Limbic are also assign emotional evaluations, such as anger, fear, sadness and joy to the events that occur. There is also a portion of the Limbic area that creates attachments. It is important to realize that there is no moral judgment in the Limbic Brain.

THOUGHT - CORTEX

The CORTEX is the outer layer of the brain. It is also known as the Cerebral Cortex. It provides for the functions of thinking, imagining and creating. The Cortex is interconnected to the other brain regions. When it is functioning in a healthy way, it provides integration and executive controls over the lower layers of the brain. Morality, judgment, reasoning and logic are all brought into the evaluation process by a mature, healthy Cortex. Neurogenesis, the growth and development of new neurons, and neuroplasticity, the rewiring of neural circuits, each take place regularly in the cortical regions of the brain.

This region, although designed to execute control and integration over the lower brain layers can be shut down when too much limbic activity provides dopamine levels so high that they damage the connections to the Cortex and the pleasure seeking drive becomes so great that it takes the Cortex offline. The result is behavior that is strictly devoid of logic, reasoning and good judgment. As mentioned above, fear and anxiety can also shut down the Cortex. This is one of the reasons pornographers combine gore and violence with nudity.

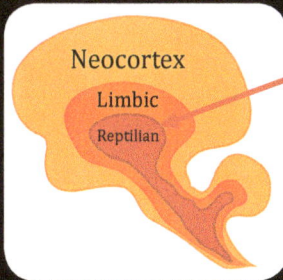

The Reptilian Brain
SURVIVAL

Anxiety, fear, and other stresses can allow this part to **shut down** the other parts of the brain.

*Do not let your hearts be **troubled** or **afraid**. . . John 14:27*

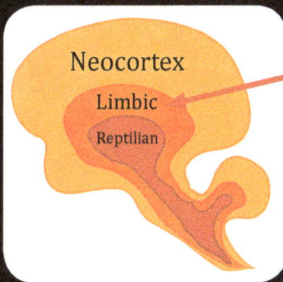

(Diagram labels: Neocortex, Limbic, Reptilian)

The Limbic Brain
GRATIFICATION

Seeks dopamine . . .
Responds to desires . . .

There is no moral judgment in the limbic brain.

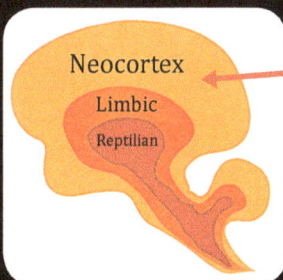

(Diagram labels: Neocortex, Limbic, Reptilian)

The Neocortex Brain
THOUGHT

Logic, reasoning, morality . . .
Good judgement, virtues . . .

. . .if there is anything worthy of praise, think about these things. Phil 4:8

(Diagram labels: Neocortex, Limbic, Reptilian)

THE ADOLESCENT BRAIN

Amazing new technologies have allowed scientists to learn more about the growth of the brain and to investigate the connections between brain function, development, and behavior. Remarkable insights on brain maturation have altered former assumptions.

The belief for many years was that the volume of gray matter was at its highest in very early childhood, and gradually declined as a child grew. Today's technology revealed that the high point of the volume of gray matter occurs during early adolescence. Throughout childhood, the volume of gray matter in the Cortex increases and then declines. The Cortex, which is responsible for thought and reasoning, develops during the pre-teen years. Since decline in volume is the sign of maturation into an adult brain, these findings push the timeline of brain maturity into adolescence and young adulthood.

Technology scans also lead scientists to believe that different parts of the Cortex mature at different rates. Those areas concerned with basic functions mature first. (Such as those parts used to process information from the senses and those that control movement.). The parts of the brain in control of more executive control, those accountable for adult behavior, are among the last to mature. (Such as those parts responsible for impulse control and planning ahead.)

Some people misinterpret this information and think teens are not capable of executive control until they are in their twenties. Think of the development of a teen's arm muscles. If two boys start out with the same size biceps and one lifts weights and works on developing his muscles, he will have more strength than the one who does not work out. It is the same with the brain. The development of the executive part of his brain (Cortex) will be determined by the activities, thoughts and actions, done during his teen years.

Thus, the greater potential for forming habitual behaviors exists in the brain of a teenager. That is why establishing good, healthy behaviors during the years the brain is pruning itself is so important. It also means the younger a person is when exposed to pornography the more easily formed are the neural pathways to compulsion and addiction. These images will generally have a greater impact on a teen brain than that of a mature adult. It is why the warnings "for adult audiences only" are on movies. (However, pornography is poison to the brain of anyone!)

This growth in maturity starts when a child is young. Think about the brain of an infant. The baby brain is operating out of the Reptilian Brain and the Limbic Brain. The baby will be "responding" to stimuli. The Cortex is not in control. If hungry, the response to that feeling is to cry. If wet, the same response. As the baby grows and language is learned, there will be a gradual increase of personal control. By the time youngsters are being potty trained, we refer to them as being a "Big Boy" or "Big Girl" when they can exhibit the ability to make the decision to use the toilet instead of a diaper. This process is showing development in the Cortex. They are now showing "control" with using the Cortex Brain and not just "responding" to the Limbic Brain. Your teen will need to intentionally strengthen the Cortex part of the brain to be in charge of the Limbic Brain.

A very simple tool for bringing attention to this necessity is to literally ask your child to evaluate their decisions by identifying if he is using his "Baby Brain" and just responding to a feeling or if he is using his "Big Boy Brain" and controlling his feelings with proper actions or using his "Grownup Brain" and showing mature behavior. The goal is to strengthen the Cortex and guide your child's maturation in using his "Grown Up Brain." It is not that on your child's 24th birthday he suddenly has a mature adult brain. It needs to be exercised in order to reach maturity. Those who are caught up in the world of pornography and masturbation often have arrested growth and even though they are adults, will function with the brain of an adolescent.

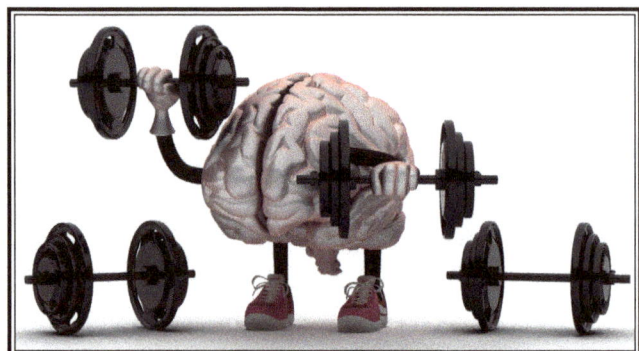

HOW TO APPROACH YOUR CHILD

DON'T DESPAIR

With a basic understanding of the brain science behind your child's struggle with pornography and how habits are both formed and unformed, you're ready to learn how to approach your teen and begin using practical tools and solutions to help him start down the path to breaking free.

Discovering that your child is involved with pornography can induce feelings of panic, fear, and even hopelessness, which may cause you to overreact and approach the situation in ways that may not be helpful or productive. To help combat these unhelpful reactions, remind yourself that every situation and child is different. It's impossible to know or predict exactly how exposure to pornography will affect each person. Be careful to avoid making assumptions, jumping to conclusions, or declaring, "All is lost!" Children are incredibly resourceful and resilient, and with your faith, love and support there isn't anything they can't get through. Don't despair, there is great hope! Countless struggling individuals all over the world have found this path to healing, and the success stories are common and far too numerous to count.

Don't Try it Alone:

Please remember that as a parent, you don't have to do this alone. You have a Father in Heaven who loves you and loves your child. You have the power of Our Lord, Jesus Christ to assist you. You can and should call upon the Holy Trinity for grace. Before you talk with your son, offer a heart-felt prayer and ask for the guidance of the Holy Spirit. In Luke 12:12 we're promised, *"For the Holy Spirit will teach you at that moment what you should say."* Be sensitive and open to the Holy's Spirit's promptings and insights during your conversation with your child. In the Blessed Virgin Mary, you also have a Mother in heaven who is the perfect human example of complete cooperation with God's plan in her life and who longs to intercede for you. You have the example of her husband, St. Joseph, a pillar of purity and one who understands the challenges of protecting a child from the dangers of the world. You can call upon the intercession of the saints who faced temptations of the flesh during their lifetime and now, though departed in body, work in spirit to build up the Kingdom of God.

TIPS FOR APPROACHING YOUR TEEN

In their book, Parenting with Grace, Gregory K. Popcak, Ph.D., and his wife Lisa, offer the following insight: "Learning about God's creation and using it in the manner God intended is one aspect of what Catholics call "natural law." Catholics are able to use faith and reason to raise the kind of children God would have us raise for Him. Today, both parents and professionals can have a clearer picture than ever about what the "Book of Nature" says about the kind of parenting methods that lead to healthier brain development, stronger moral reasoning, and a deeper capacity for intimacy and empathy in our children. Catholic parents are encouraged by the Church to learn everything they can about creating the conditions that allow their child's brain, body and spirit to develop to their full, godly potential."[16]

Every child and every family has its own unique personality, characteristics and background—everyone is different, so there's no perfect script for talking with your child about their pornography use. However, other families have found that the general guidelines found on the following pages often help.

Note: Even if a teen refuses to talk about the issue, or rebels against doing anything to stop their porn use, continue to be patient, kind and unconditionally loving. Look for natural opportunities to implement any or all of the following guidelines. And no matter what, never give up!

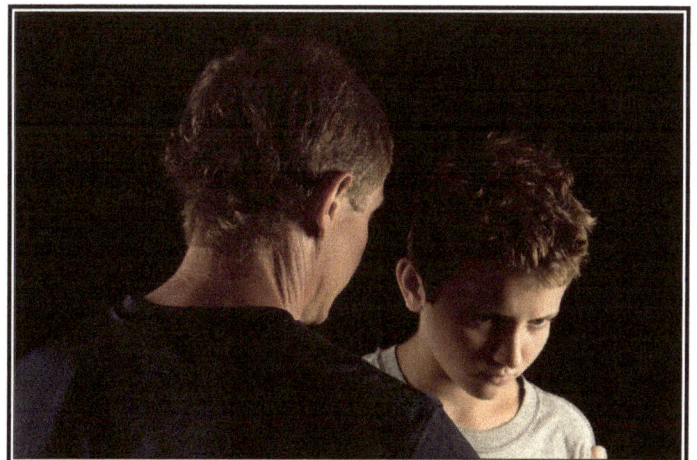

Practice the Art of True Empathy: Your first inclination may be to express anger or disappointment, give a lecture, or conduct an interrogation. Instead, set aside all your pre-conceived notions, your own feelings and agenda, and just open your heart to what your child is telling you. Have a deep yearning to truly understand what he is feeling and going through. Try to get into the space where his experience becomes more relevant than your own; where you strive to step into his shoes and see the world through his eyes. Again, call upon God and ask for the Holy Spirit to help you practice the art of true empathy. Remember, this communication time is not about what he has or hasn't done. It's an opportunity to discover who your child is as a person, his views and deepest feelings, his concerns and insights. It's also an opportunity to allow your child to get to know you. For both of you, it can be a powerful time to explore and discover more about one another.

Separate Your Child From Their Behavior: In 1 Samuel 16:7 we read, "Do not judge from his appearance or from his lofty stature, because I have rejected him. Not as man sees does God see, because man sees the appearance but the LORD looks into the heart." In order to enjoy real, open communication, it's important that your child knows that you love him for who he is, regardless of his behaviors. It's essential that you see his true self completely separate from his behaviors. Even though he may pretend otherwise, your teen is still very dependent on your opinion of him and craves your acceptance and validation. Scientific studies show that the most powerful communication we share as human beings are the unconscious, and non-verbal signals of what we think and feel about each other. You may say the words, but if you aren't sincere, your teen will sense it, and it will create a chasm between you. As you talk, remind yourself how much you love your child. This love will show in your eyes as you maintain eye contact, and in your warm and open body language and posture.

Ask Non-Judgmental Questions: Before you ask a question, ask yourself, "How will knowing the answer to this help me help my child?" Try to make sure that your questions are not self-serving, passive-aggressive or leading in any way. Ask simple, direct questions that allow you to understand and gather helpful information, without allowing your emotions to get the best of you.

For example, you might inquire:

- When did you first start looking at pornography?

- Where do you go to view it?

- What kinds of feelings do you have while you're viewing it and afterward?

- How can I help you?

Give Validation: After your son has expressed all that he needs to about his feelings and what he's been going through, it's your turn. You may be a bit shocked by what you've heard, and you may not know how to respond. That's perfectly normal. Assure your son of your unconditional love for him, and that you will be there for him no matter what. If he feels your love and support he will be far more willing to continue down the healing path with you.

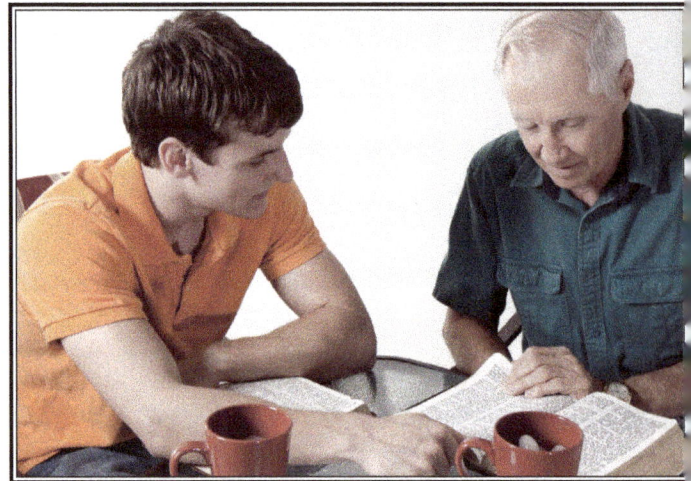

Teach the Brain Science: People who are involved with pornography typically fall into three primary categories:

- They don't understand why pornography use is such a big deal and make light of any suggestions that there's anything wrong with it.

- They realize that pornography is harmful and contrary to God's sacred plan, but they're in denial about their own personal struggles with it, and/or they keep trying to hide the extent of their porn use or keep it a secret altogether.

- They feel a tremendous burden of shame; they feel trapped, weak, and broken. They've tried to break free and keep failing. They feel hopeless.

In any of these cases, your child will gain tremendous insight, understanding and benefit when you teach him about the brain science behind his pornography use. This will help those who are complacent to take the issue seriously; those in denial to come to grips with the truth about their struggles; and those buried in shame to realize how they've been manipulated and set up by the porn industry—that they're not a loser or a lost cause, and that there is a rational, logical, and scientific explanation behind their struggles.

Teach the Sacredness of God's Plan for Sexuality: Avoid confusing messages like, "Sex is evil and dirty, but be sure and save it for someone you really care about!" Avoid the dark, sterile and body-parts-centered view of sex that Hollywood, many sex-education programs, and pornographers portray. Instead, teach the sacredness of God's plan for sexuality—a beautiful, wonderful, and powerful gift to look forward to at the right time with the right person in marriage. At all costs avoid causing your child to feel shameful about his sexuality—sexual shame is one of the primary contributing factors that can lead to pornography addiction and lifelong unhealthy sexual behaviors. The "*Funnel of Love*" vs. the "*Funnel of Lust*" can be very helpful in this discussion.

Teach Youth They Can "Bridle" This Sacred Power: Telling a teen not to feel attracted toward the opposite sex or never to feel arousal is like telling a cloud not to rain. These powerful feelings are built into every cell of his body, are part of his genetic make-up, and are given to him by God. Teaching him to deny these feelings or telling him they are evil not only rejects the gift God has given us, it creates shame and often drives teens to act out sexually. Instead, teach him that he can bridle his passions and attractions and use them in the time and place for which they were created.

The rider of a powerful horse does not permit the horse to run wild, unrestrained and without controls. Doing so places the rider in great peril. Rather, the rider uses reins

attached to a bridle to harness and direct the horse's power for productive and positive purposes. A skilled horseman knows when to hold the animal back, when to turn it loose, and how to direct it along desired paths, to arrive at the destination. We must become similarly skilled in harnessing the power of our sexuality.

Teach your son that these stirrings he feels are normal and good, and have been placed within him by God for very special and sacred purposes. Rather than denying and completely shutting these feelings down, teach your son about his power to bridle, control and direct these sacred powers in healthy and appropriate ways. Taking the reins, he can travel the pathways of proper dating relationships, courtship and eventually marriage. At the right time and place, united with the love of his life in the sacred bonds of marriage, he can experience the exhilarating and beautiful full expression of his sexual energy in loving a spouse. Sexual energy does not always have to be expressed genitally. There are times, even in marriage, when that will not be possible. The true power of sexual energy is to give of oneself. Harnessing that energy in service to an individual, family or organization is a healthy way of expressing and releasing it. If he has a calling from God for the celibate life, this training will also help prepare him for that vocation.

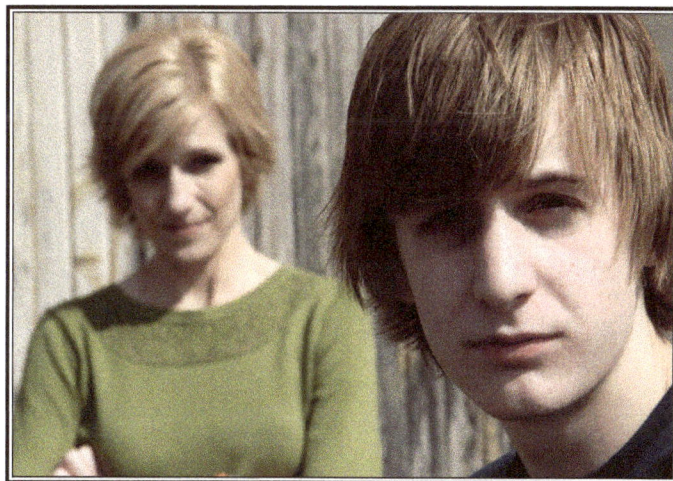

Help Youth Clearly Identify Their "Why?": We form our most dominant attitudes and mental models based on the people and things that have deep meaning for us. When teaching your son about healthy and appropriate sexuality, help him clearly identify his deepest motives— <u>why</u> he should avoid pornography and wait until marriage to have sexual relations. Using negative motivations like "You'll become addicted!" "You could get an STD!" "You might get pregnant!" "God will punish you!" is ineffective with teens. One of the problems with this approach is that most teens believe they are indestructible—"That won't happen to me!" They're often so focused on the here and now, they disregard the consequences and think, "I'll worry about that later."

Brain studies on human motivation clearly show that teenagers naturally will gravitate toward a positive motive over avoiding a negative one. Do you have to make a child stop dawdling and force them to run from one exciting amusement park ride to the next? Do you have to threaten a group of young athletes to clean off the patio so they can play basketball? How about lecturing a high school senior about personal appearance so she'll spend four highly focused hours preparing for the prom? When something has deep meaning, teens are highly motivated and self-governing. Here's an exercise you can use to help your son identify some powerfully positive motives for avoiding porn and reserving the sacred gift of sexual intimacy for marriage.

Exercise #8: The Gift

Find an appropriate time to guide your teen through this process. Ask your child to write down thoughts and feelings in response to the following instructions and questions. Note: You may find that this works well even with a group of teens together.

- Visualize in your mind your perfect future spouse. Describe his or her characteristics in detail. Describe the kinds of choices that person is making right now.

- What is the best way to find your perfect spouse? If you have identified the qualities you are looking for in a spouse, it could be assumed that your future spouse would be looking for those same qualities in you! By developing those same values, goals, choices etc. in yourself, you would be attractive to the type of person you want to marry!

- Imagine you are standing at the marriage altar looking into the beautiful eyes of your beloved. Knowing you have saved yourself for him or her (the most precious gift you can bring to that sacred altar), how does that make your new spouse feel? How do you feel?

CAUTION: Please remember, there are some teens who have made mistakes. DO NOT shame them with this exercise. Stress the fact that they can move forward right now and make the right choices. As they visualize standing at the marriage altar, they can think, "I remember the day I committed to save this sacred gift for this special person. From that day forward I did it!"

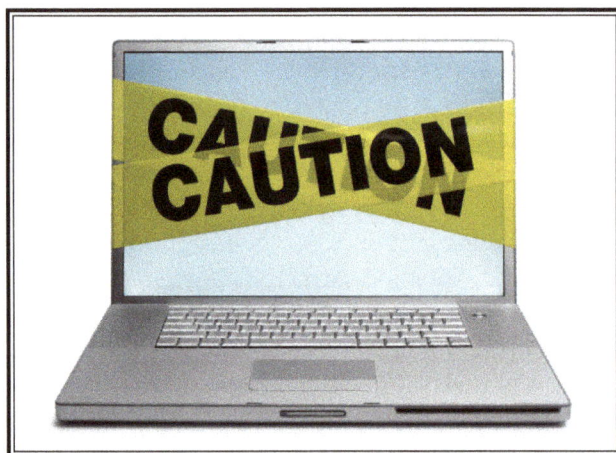

Map Out a Plan Together: Recognize that your child needs your help—he can't break free without you. He needs to have confidence that you're on his side and willing to fight this thing with him no matter what. As you work as a team to map out a plan of action, consider the following priorities:

Put Protections in Place: Help your son understand that in order for him to start the healing process, he needs to be protected from the sinister attacks of pornographers. As you consider with him the various outlets where he typically looks at pornography, discuss the protections you can put in place. For example: Internet filters and accountability software on computers, tablets, or cell phones; parental controls on gaming systems or cable TV; moving computers out of bedrooms into a public traffic place in the home; and set aside certain hours where Internet and other media are made unavailable. Keep in mind that it may be necessary for a time to shut down all Internet access. Talk openly and honestly with each other in a loving and trusting way and come up with a Protection Plan.

Ask What He Thinks: Ask your son what he specifically plans to do to stop viewing pornography and how you can help. You may be surprised at how clearly he recognizes where he needs the most help and what boundaries should be put into place. Lovingly give any additional ideas you feel would be helpful. It's important that you don't try to force your way of thinking, but simply offer guidance and suggestions. If you rule with an iron fist and manage to shut down all porn portals in the home, he'll likely rebel and find ways to get access elsewhere.

Replacement Activities: In many cases, a child engages in unwanted behaviors because of boredom or a lack of truly fulfilling activities that validate his self-esteem, creativity, abilities and talents. You can be instrumental in involving him in activities that provide learning and growth; that create purpose in his life such as: service opportunities, faith practices, hobbies, art, music, sports, acting, fishing, outdoor skills, education, business skills, computer skills, getting a job, etc. Find out what he's good at, and help him open new opportunities. He needs to refocus this sexual energy into healthy outlets.

Caution—Be careful not to dictate or push what you think he should pursue. You can offer suggestions, but allow him to make the choice. Also, don't overload your son by filling up every waking moment with activities. He needs downtime. The stress of too much going on can actually push him to seek escape through sexual outlets.

Additional factors: It's also important to note that your child may be struggling with other things besides unwanted sexual behaviors. In fact, these behaviors may just be a symptom of other issues. It could be a childhood trauma, attention and impulsivity issues, depression, anxiety, mood problems or an inability to attach. If your child is experiencing severe behavior problems that are in addition to the unwanted sexual behaviors, or if he is

not making any forward progress with overcoming the sexual behaviors, it may be an indication that you need some additional professional and specialized help.

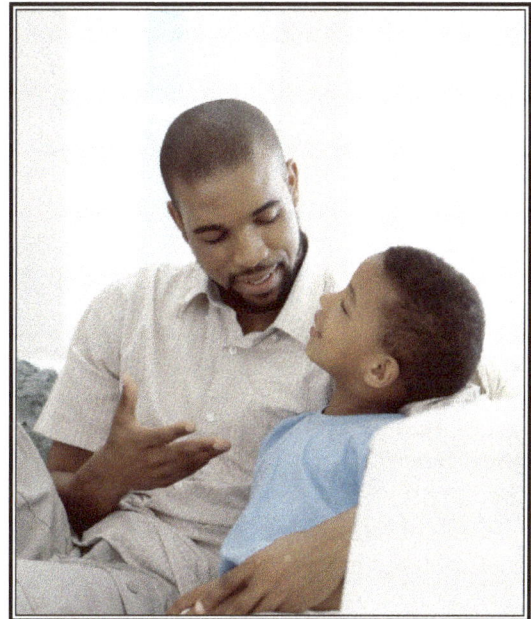

Exercise #9: The Talk

Think back to when you were a kid and any experiences you had with your parents and "The Talk." How did your parents talk with you about sexuality? How did their approach make you feel? Now that you are a parent, what do you think they could have done to improve their approach? *(Complete this exercise in your private journal.)*

Exercise #10: Create a Script and Schedule a Time

How have you approached the issue of sexuality with your son up to this point? Without telling him about your plan, schedule a regular time on your personal calendar as a reminder to talk with your son about these things. This will help you continue the conversation until it becomes more comfortable and natural, and you no longer wish to avoid it.

Write out a script or set of notes in advance for what you will say and the points you want to cover. If you need some ideas and suggestions in this area, please see the appendix in this guidebook for suggestions of additional resources. *(Complete this exercise in your private journal.)*

BREAKING FREE

As a parent, it is vital that you understand you cannot shame or demand your child change. Unhealthy sexual behavior already has trapped him in sin and shame. To become free, parents may want to tell their child to just avoid the temptation and use willpower to stay pure. Although that advice sounds correct, it really is not enough. Using this approach leads to the avoidance cycle and eventual failure. You must lead your son with unconditional love and teach proven tools for freedom.

AVOIDANCE AND WILLPOWER ARE NOT ENOUGH

What happens when you try to force a thought out of your mind? For instance, right now I don't want you to think about a big, bright, pink elephant. No matter what, DO NOT think about that elephant! Of course, the more you try to fight and keep the image out of your mind, the more it forces its way in. In fact, you may not have been thinking of a pink elephant until you read about it here, but now it is all you are thinking about! In psychology, this is called an *intrusive thought.* Continually attempting to force the same intrusive thoughts, urges or feelings out of your mind can hopelessly plunge you into the *Avoidance Cycle.*

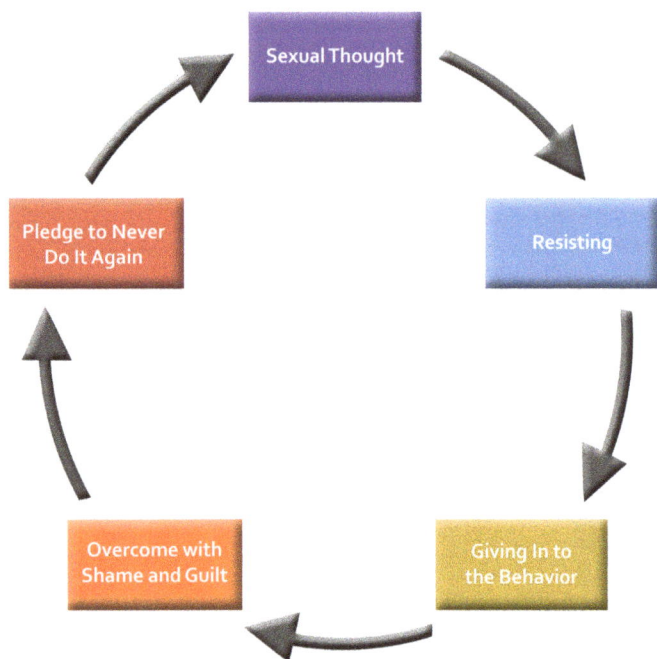

THE AVOIDANCE CYCLE

When teenagers try to overcome pornography use, the most common strategy they use to break out is "Avoidance and Willpower." For example, when a typical teen starts feeling the urge to look at porn, he immediately goes to war with the thought, trying to force it out of his mind. He reasons, "I've got to avoid sexual thoughts at all costs." He grits his teeth, clinches his fists and uses sheer willpower to keep the thoughts and urges at bay.

What happens when he tries to force the sexual thoughts and urges out of his mind? They drill their way in with even more power, until they become "intrusive." Often he fights for as long as he can, and then finally worn out by the battle, he gives in. With pornography and masturbation, this is a very common scenario. The teen fights the urges for hours, days, weeks or even months and then, finally exhausted, gives in.

As he views the images, powerful neurochemicals flood the brain, and there is a very temporary but highly satisfying relief from the battle. "Finally, I don't have to fight these sexual thoughts and urges anymore!" he thinks. However, once the chemicals dissipate from his brain, logic and reasoning return, and then guilt, regret and shame set in. The teen makes a new vow to fight the urge, and the whole "Avoidance Cycle" starts all over again. People can be stuck in this cycle for years. "So," you might be thinking, "If avoidance and sheer willpower are not the answer, what is?"

Through repetition over time, your son has built a specific habit and brain circuitry that has him trapped in pornography use. Because his brain is "neuroplastic," meaning it is highly moldable and changeable, he can learn to use a technique called **"C-IT"** as a way to shrink his porn addiction circuitry and replace it with new healthy sexuality circuitry. How? Through consistent repetition over time—the same way he originally built his porn habit. The same type of process that got him into this mess can get him out!

Ask God to give you the courage to seek out biblical principles. Encourage your teen to turn to Christ to understand how to respond to the temptations.

JESUS CHRIST GAVE US THE KEY TO FREEDOM!

No trial has come to you but what is human. God is faithful and will not let you be tried beyond your strength; but with the trial he will also provide a way out, so that you may be able to bear it. 1 Corinthians 10:13

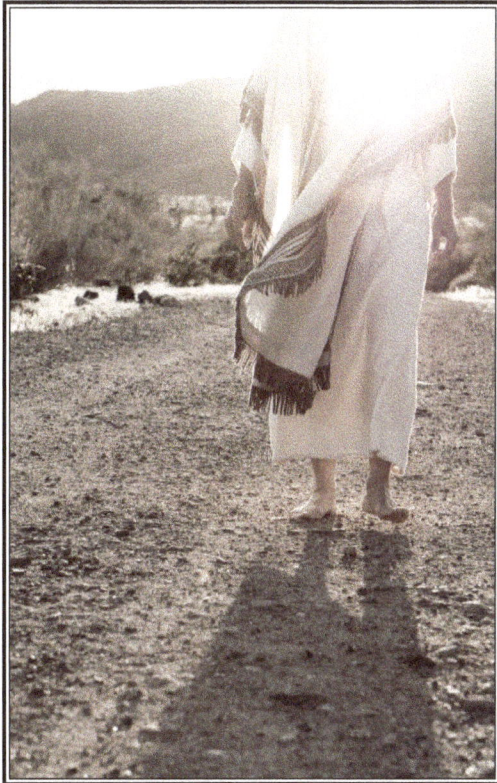

Jesus' response to the temptations of the devil recorded in **Matthew, Chapter 4** gives us direction.

Then Jesus was led by the Spirit into the desert to be tempted by the devil. He fasted for forty days and forty nights, and afterwards he was hungry. The tempter approached and said to him, "If you are the Son of God, command that these stones become loaves of bread." He said in reply, "It is written: 'One does not live by bread alone, but by every word that comes forth from the mouth of God.'"

Then the devil took him to the holy city, and made him stand on the parapet of the temple, and said to him, "If you are the Son of God, throw yourself down. For it is written: 'He will command his angels concerning you' and 'with their hands they will support you, lest you dash your foot against a stone.'"

Jesus answered him, "Again it is written, 'You shall not put the Lord, your God, to the test.'" Then the devil took him up to a very high mountain, and showed him all the kingdoms of the world in their magnificence, and he said to him, "All these I shall give to you, if you will prostrate yourself and worship me."

At this, Jesus said to him, "Get away, Satan! It is written: 'The Lord, your God, shall you worship and him alone shall you serve.'" Then the devil left him and, behold, angels came and ministered to him.

———————————————

After Jesus had fasted 40 days, Satan came tempting Him. Why then? Because Satan perceived Jesus to be at His weakest point—physically exhausted, hungry, thirsty, etc. This is when Satan comes tempting teens; when they're "B.L.H.A.S.T.ed"—(Bored or Burned Out; Lonely; Hungry; Angry, Anxious or Afraid; Stressed or Tired).

When sexual temptation hits a teenager, his typical response is probably to either:

A. Give in, or

B. Try to use sheer willpower (the white-knuckle approach) to resist and avoid the temptation. As outlined above, this response traps the teen in the "Avoidance Cycle."

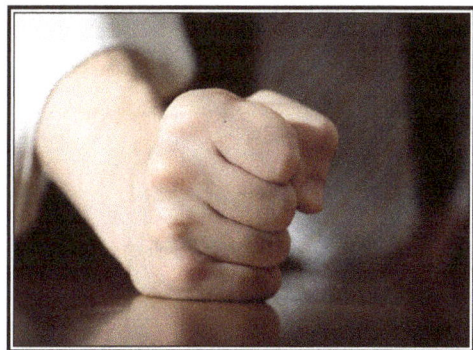

Rather than "Option A" or "Option B" — which both result in "giving in" to the temptation — Jesus chose a completely different response.

He fasted for forty days and forty nights, and afterwards he was hungry. The tempter approached and said to him, "If you are the Son of God, command that these stones become loaves of bread." (Matthew 4: 2-3)

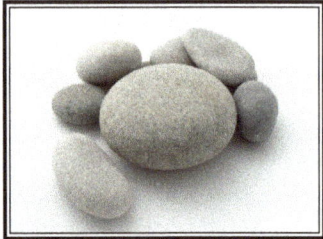

Why does the Scripture tell us that Jesus was hungry? Of course he was hungry—he had just fasted for forty days and nights. The comment on Jesus' physical hunger reminds us of two things:

Jesus' humanity: Despite the fact that he was God, Jesus experienced the same physical urges we do—including hunger. We might be tempted to shrug off Jesus' reaction to temptation with the claim, "Of course he avoided it, he was God—he doesn't really understand what it's like!" This Scripture reminds us that Jesus <u>does</u> understand, and his response can help us as well.

The power of the temptation: This reminder of Jesus' physical hunger serves as the foundation for his temptation. It's as if Satan is saying, "Jesus, you're hungry and exhausted. Look at that stone over there on the ground—doesn't it look like a loaf of bread? Give in to your appetite. Use your power to transform the stone and relieve your hunger pains."

Confronted with this temptation, most of us would probably close our eyes, grit our teeth and attempt to force the thought of bread out of our minds—"I won't think about bread, I won't, I won't!" Jesus didn't fear, give in, run or avoid. He chose a different response—one that was effective 2,000 years ago, and, as the latest brain research and clinical experience show, is just as effective today.

Satan attempted to create doubt in the Savior's mind with the statement, "If you are the Son of God . . .." But Jesus held fast to His **true identity** and with boldness faced the tempter head-on. He **exposed the lie** and then **announced the truth** by declaring the words of His Father:

"It is written: 'One does not live by bread alone, but by every word that comes forth from the mouth of God.'" (Matthew 4:4)

Three times Jesus was tempted, and each time he followed the same process—He:

CLAIMED His true identity;

CONFRONTED the lie; and

CORRECTED the lie with the truth. Finally, after the tempter gave up and left him, Jesus

CONNECTED with others—He went about teaching, lifting up, loving, and serving.

We call that the Christ Approach: "C-It".

From that time on, Jesus began to preach and say; "Repent, for the kingdom of heaven is at hand." Matthew 4:17

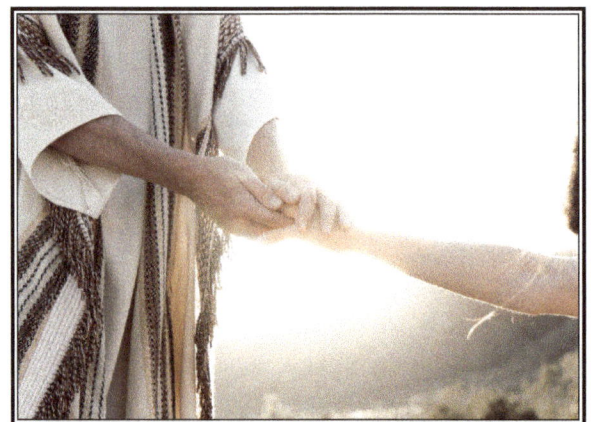

THE "C-IT" PROCESS

Your child can follow Jesus' example, use the same process to effectively fight Satan's temptation, and begin breaking free from pornography use.

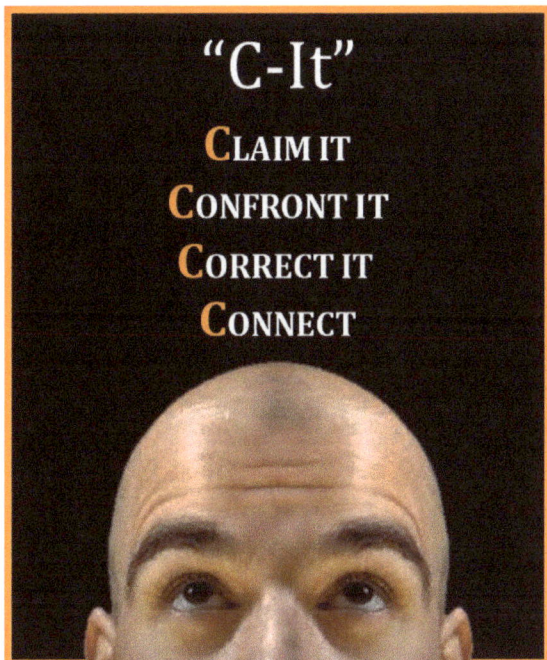

"C-It"

CLAIM IT
CONFRONT IT
CORRECT IT
CONNECT

CLAIM Christ and Your True Identity:

When your son feels the urge or temptation to look at pornography, the first thing he should do is say a prayer asking for the Holy Spirit's help and thinking of Jesus Christ—imagine His face; hear His voice; feel Him standing nearby.

In that frame of mind, your son then thinks about his own true identity—"I am a child of God. He loves me and has a wonderful mission and purpose for me on this earth. I feel the Holy Spirit here with me. I am a child of God with dignity and worth beyond measure. (Encourage your child to say these things out loud if possible. If he's in a public place where that isn't appropriate, he can whisper them to himself or say them in his mind.)

It's no coincidence that the account of Jesus' temptation comes immediately after Jesus' baptism in the River Jordan by John the Baptist. After the baptism, we read:

And a voice came from the heavens, saying, "This is my beloved Son, with whom I am well pleased." (Matthew 3:17)

The very next verse is the beginning of his temptation:

"Then Jesus was led by the Spirit into the desert to be tempted by the devil." (Matthew 4:1)

Jesus was able to hold fast to his identity as the Son of God in the face of temptation because God had just affirmed His identity. Give your child this same gift of affirmation so that he can hold tight to it in the face of temptation. Spend time talking with your child about his identity. Make a conscious effort to regularly affirm in your child his identity as your "beloved son" and his dignity as a member of the Body of Christ and beloved son of God. If he doesn't know who he is, he can't know God's plan and purpose for his life. His view of himself can have a profound effect on everyday living.

CONFRONT the Lie:

The sexual urge or temptation will always be based on a lie. Satan is the "father of all lies" and uses falsehoods to deceive and manipulate sons and daughters of God into doing his will. Your son needs to identify the lie and expose it, out loud if possible. For example, some lies might be:

"You feel stressed and pornography is a way to feel better." (But it only works for a short time. In the end it makes things worse.)

"You need pornography. You can't make it without it." (No one has ever died by not seeing pornography or masturbating!)

"You're going to give in eventually, so you may as well go ahead and look." (You can claim victory and not give in to the lure of pornography!)

These are lies planted in the mind by the tempter. As these thoughts pass through your child's mind, he needs to confront it and declare, "This is a lie. All of these things are a lie. The Devil is a liar." Again, out loud if possible, and if not, your son should shout them in his mind.

Exercise #11: Identify Satan's Lies

Together, you and your child need to make a list of the lies that Satan and the pornographers want him to believe. He may need your assistance in recognizing the lies about sexuality because your son has grown up in a society that has promoted these lies as truth.

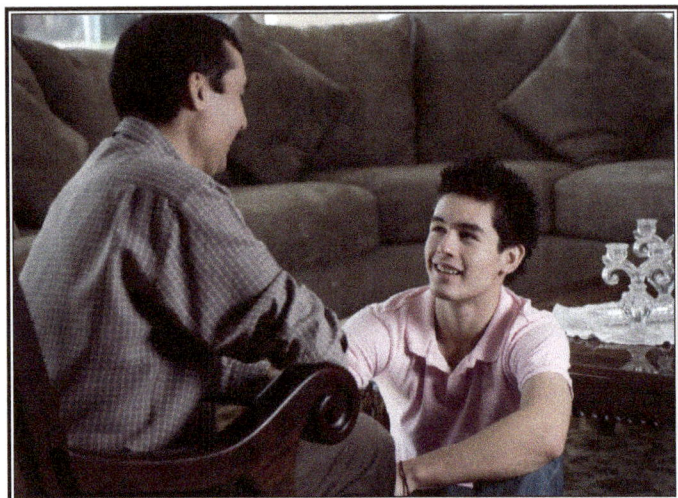

As a parent who grew up in this same sex-saturated society, you may also struggle with recognizing the lies! *(See pages 41-44 for more information on the truth of God's plan. Study Theology of the Body, talk to a priest or spiritual director. Contact Elizabeth Ministry International for suggested readings etc.)*

CORRECT by stating the truth:

After the first two steps, your son needs to immediately correct the lie with a statement of truth —"The porn might feel good for a few minutes, but afterward I will feel like garbage! That's what always happens! I don't need pornography. I have the Holy Spirit. I have the love of Jesus. I have my guardian angel and the support of the Communion of Saints. I have my parents and my friends. I have so many blessings and things I'm grateful for. I don't have to give in, because I have the power of Christ and the Holy Spirit with me. Get away Satan!" Your child can quote memorized scripture that is special to him, prayers and powerful quotes. He should continue to "announce the truth" until he feels the urge leaving him.

Exercise #12 Truth Statements

Help your child prepare for this step by seeking out scripture passages and prayers to memorize. Together find quotes that proclaim the truth. Sharing stories from the lives of the saints will help identify quotes and life belief statements.

CONNECT with or serve someone:

Satan seeks to keep us separated and isolated from our true self, from God, and from others. He's like a wolf trying to separate us from the herd, get us off alone, and then devour us. (Help your son remember that Christ always comes after us—even leaving the 99 sheep to seek after the one. Matthew 18:12) Your son should look for an immediate way to connect with his true self, God or another person.

There are many ways to do this connecting. Here are some suggestions:

Encourage your son to connect with his true self by:
- Engaging in a favorite hobby.
- Doing an athletic event like jogging.

Encourage your son to connect with God by:
- Listening to uplifting music.
- Journaling letters to God (and God's response).
- Attending a religious service or youth event.
- Engaging in prayer.

Encourage your son to connect with others by:
- Volunteering for a charitable organization.
- Sending a text or making a call to encourage a friend or family member.
- Visiting an elderly relative or neighbor.
- Doing a chore for a family member.
- Smiling at a stranger.

The key is to come out of isolation and make a connection with an activity or person that is enjoyable and meaningful.

Teach your child to stop in a tempting situation and look at what CHRIST did! He used the four "C" words:

Claim - Confront - Correct - Connect

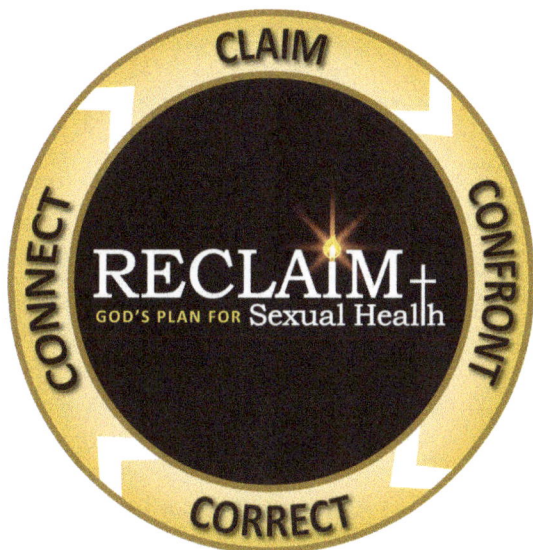

While "C-IT" is a simple tool, it isn't something that just happens automatically. When an urge hits your teen, his brain is going to default to porn unless he interrupts that habit and purposely moves himself into the "C-IT" process. Help him practice the "C - It" steps so it becomes his automatic response.

THE "C-IT" PROCESS TAKES PREPARATION AND PRACTICE!

To become skilled in the "C-IT" technique, your teen needs to prepare and practice. Here are some tips that will help:

Create a Script in Advance: You can help your son create a "C-IT" script in advance. Talk about the most common urges he faces, and help him write out a script for each situation. Then, he can carry it with him on a 3x5 card, or on his cell phone, and pull it out when needed. For success, his mind has to have practiced a "C-IT" script over and over so that it forms a habitual response.

Practice, Practice, Practice! Role play with your son and have him imagine a situation where he's feeling the urge to look at pornography. You can rattle off the "lies" that Satan typically plants in his mind, and he can use his script to respond. If your child is uncomfortable doing this with you, he can do the role playing and practicing on his own.

Exercise #13: Help Your Child Create a "C-IT" Script

Sit down with your child and review the training for the "C-IT" technique. Be sure to read the verses in Matthew, chapter four, and discuss how Jesus gave us the example for this powerful tool. Help your son create his first "C-IT" script, and then do a role play so he can practice responding to an urge. This will also work with other temptations!

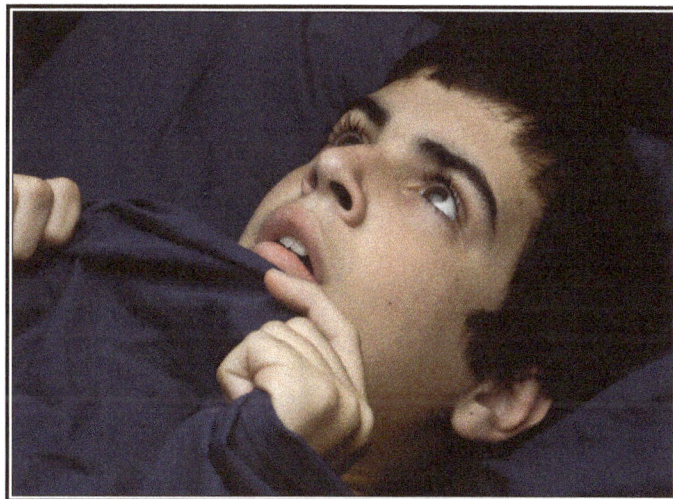

Special Note: When the "urge" starts washing over your teen like a giant wave, he may not be able to think clearly enough to use the "C-IT" technique. A powerful tool that can help him calm his brain and invite the Holy Spirit to be present so he can focus on "C-IT" is called "Gratitude Breathing."

This technique has been scientifically proven to calm the brain and the heart. Here's how it works—

GRATITUDE BREATHING

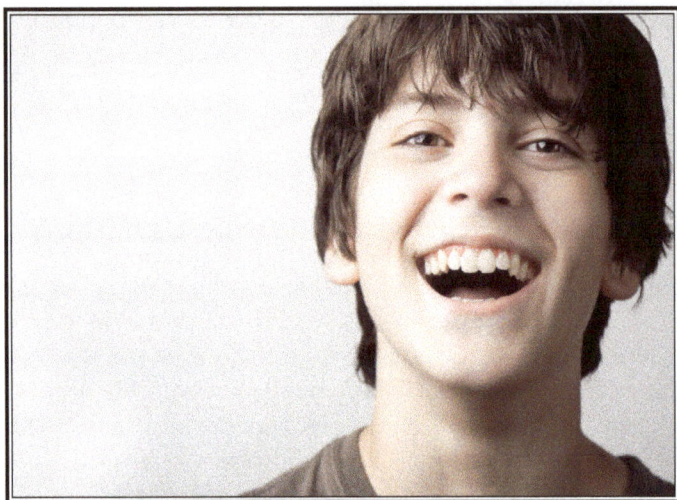

Exercise #14: Practice Gratitude Breathing

Whenever you're feeling stressed, angry, lonely or have any other negative feelings or unwanted urges, use the Gratitude Breathing technique. Become familiar with it and gain a testimony of its effectiveness. Teach it to your teen, and actually sit with your teen and do it together. Ask him how he feels afterward. Encourage him to use this technique whenever he feels the "urge" or any negative feelings sweeping over him.

Change Brain Circuitry: Help your son realize that every time he practices through role playing, he is shrinking his porn addiction circuitry and building new healthy sexuality circuitry in his brain—he is literally building a brain that over time will no longer seek pornography! The more he practices, the more quickly and deeply the brain changes will take place. This is also true every time he uses "C-IT" in real life "urge" situations. With each real life experience, he shrinks the porn habit circuitry and expands the new healthy circuitry. This is neuroplasticity at full power!

1. Take in a deep breath for a count of 6. As you're taking in the breath, imagine and feel your heart actually taking in the oxygen—visualize this. Imagine your heart is growing larger as you take in the breath. To help put the focus on your heart, you can place your hand over your heart like you do when you say the Pledge of Allegiance.

2. As you're imagining breathing oxygen into your heart, think of someone special that you are deeply grateful for—for example, your Savior, Jesus Christ. In your mind say, "I am thankful for . . . (say the person's name)" and clearly see their face. Hold their face in your mind and feel your heart filling up with gratitude for them, at the same time it's filling up with oxygen.

3. Focusing on gratitude is a wonderful way to invite the Holy Spirit to be present. Gratitude is also the emotion that has been shown to have a powerful calming effect on the brain and heart.

4. Now breathe out for a count of 6 and imagine the gratitude flowing out from your heart to fill your whole body.

5. Repeat the process as many times as needed until you feel the presence of the Holy Spirit and feel yourself calming and getting back into the "driver's seat." Now you're ready to follow the steps of the "C-IT" process.

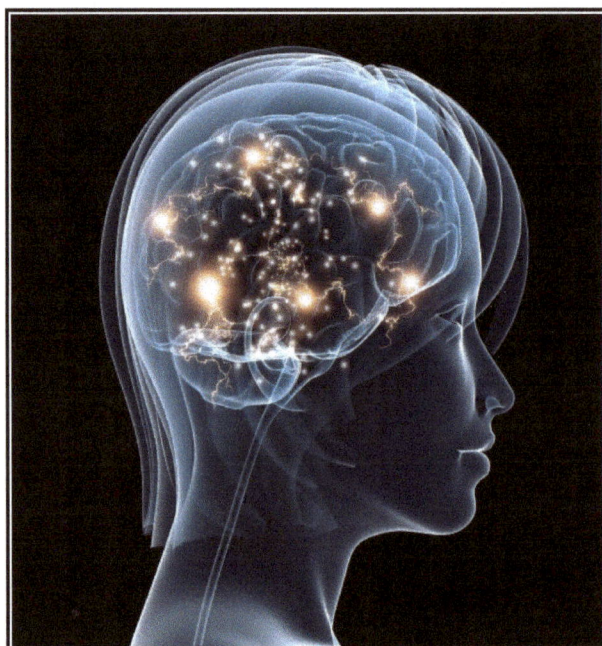

AN ADDITIONAL TOOL

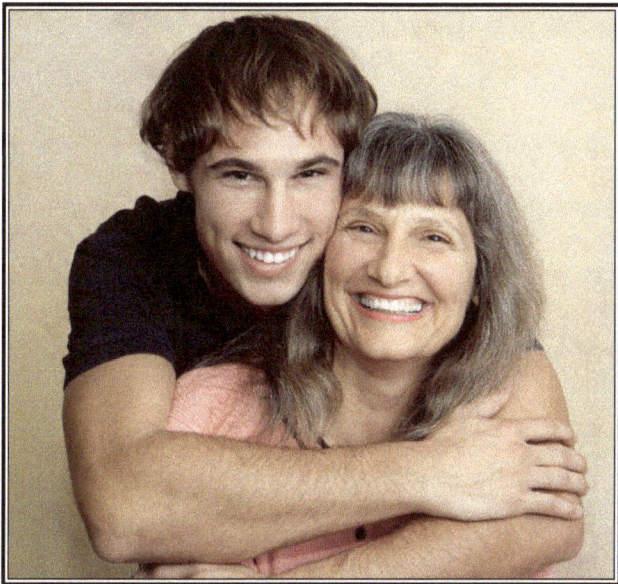

A Heart-Connection

As you seek to work with your son in overcoming pornography, you may find times when tension and conflict push you apart. Following several years of difficulty with his teenage son and the pornography issue, a father commented, "When we pass in the hall we don't say anything, we just fume at each other." A simple, yet powerful tool that has helped parents clear away their negative feelings is called a "Heart-Connection." This tool allows you as a parent to tap into your feelings of unconditional love, forgiveness, compassion and set aside ego. These powerful feelings do not originate in the brain. They must spring from the heart, then into the mind and the brain.

The heart overrides the ego-driven, self-centered brain. Communication from the heart emits an energy that is sensed by those to whom the message is intended. The power of a Heart-Connection resides in the fact that your mind cannot focus on two dissimilar thoughts at one time; it can't access two opposing attitudes at once. When your mind is dominated by negative thoughts, you can connect to your heart and replace these thoughts with positive, loving thoughts of your choosing—the light instantly dispelling the darkness.

It may surprise you how easy Heart Connections are to create and how powerful they are when implemented. Start with a blank piece of paper and an open mind. Begin by putting the name of your struggling teen (or any other family member with whom you want to improve your relationship) at the top of the page. Then make a list of all the positive attributes or things you appreciate about him. Also write down the most recent positive experience you've shared or an event that caused you to admire or feel close to your son. If you can't think of one, imagine what that kind of experience would be like, and in as much detail as possible, write it down. There it is, the beginnings of a Heart Connection.

Write the list of positive attributes and the positive experience on a 3x5 card and carry it with you. Whenever you think about your teen, or just before you're about to interact with him, connect to your heart by reviewing the contents of the card and holding them in your conscious thoughts. Don't let your son see the card or tell him what's on it. It's more powerful for him to just feel the positive energy as you hold the heart-felt thoughts in your mind.

Many parents who use this tool report back how much their teen begins to change. In actuality, with the Heart-Connection, the parent changes first and the teen naturally responds to this change. You don't see others as they are, but rather as you are. Change the way you see people, and the people you see will change. It's amazing how quickly this simple little tool begins to positively improve family relationships.

Exercise #15: Create a Heart Connection

Right now, create a simple "Heart-Connection" for your struggling son. Make sure you record it on a 3x5 card or on your phone where you can instantly and regularly access and review it. Every time you have a thought about your teen, review your Heart-Connection—on the card, your phone, or in your mind. Whenever you interact with your child, keep the words of the Heart-Connection clearly in your mind. Do this consistently, particularly before you know that you will be spending time together (i.e., just before they come home from school or before you get up in the morning) and watch the transformation unfold.

GOD IS MINDFUL OF YOU

TRUST IN GOD

Raising children in these perilous times is no easy task. In fact, it can seem downright intimidating and overwhelming. If you have a son or daughter who is struggling with pornography, we hope this Parent Primer starts you down the road of healing for both you and your child. Your whole family likely has a lot of work ahead, and it's certain that the road to recovery and healing will not always be easy.

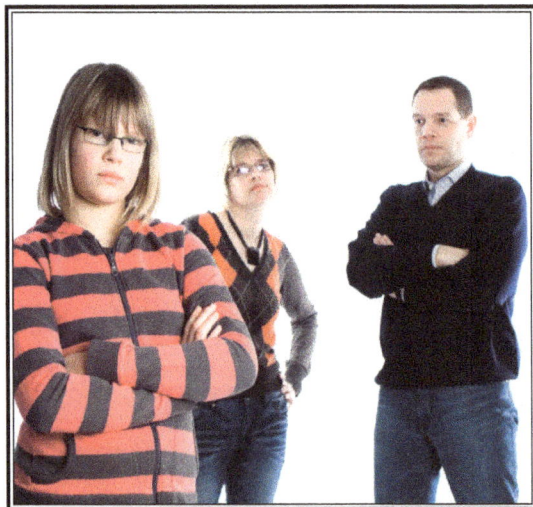

During the tough times, we are often tempted to feel hopeless or helpless. But winning the battles of life—particularly the battle to help your child reclaim God's plan for his or her sexuality—starts with believing that you are not alone in this journey. Know that God is mindful of you, your love, your devotion and your desires to help your struggling child.

In Proverbs 3:5-6 we read, *Trust in the LORD with all your heart, on your own intelligence rely not; In all your ways be mindful of Him, and He will make straight your paths.*

"For I know well the plans I have in mind for you, says the LORD, plans for your welfare, not for woe! Plans to give you a future full of hope. When you call me, when you go to pray to me, I will listen to you. When you look for me, you will find me. Yes, when you seek me with all your heart, you will find me with you, says the LORD." Jeremiah 29:11-14

Exercise #16: God's Promises

As a devoted parent who is trying to help your child reclaim God's plan for his life, take comfort in the assurance that you were blessed by God on the day of your child's Baptism to handle this and all the struggles of parenthood. Scripture is full of God's promises to parents, particularly parents who are struggling. Take some time to read through these promises and come back to them when times get tough or when you feel alone, helpless, hopeless or overwhelmed. Let the promises of the Living God wash over and comfort you.

2 Chronicles 20:15, Psalm 27:13-14,
Psalm 37:4, Psalm 55:22, Psalm 147:3,
Isaiah 49:25, Jeremiah 29:11,
John 8:36, Psalm 73:26, Romans 8:1-2,
Psalm 121:1-2, 2 Corinthians 5:17,
Psalm 103:12, Psalm 34:4-8

LOOK WITHIN

If any unhealthy sexual behavior is happening in your own life, now is the time for you to seek help and work on your own healing and recovery. The strain of facing your child's struggles will require a united effort from both parents. Elizabeth Ministry International can provide hope with an online, anonymous recovery program for adults called RECLAiM Sexual Health. The information and skills learned in this program can not only offer you help, but can also be used to teach your child. Although this program is designed for adults, many parents have used this program with their older teens. For more information, go to www.reclaimsexualhealth.com.

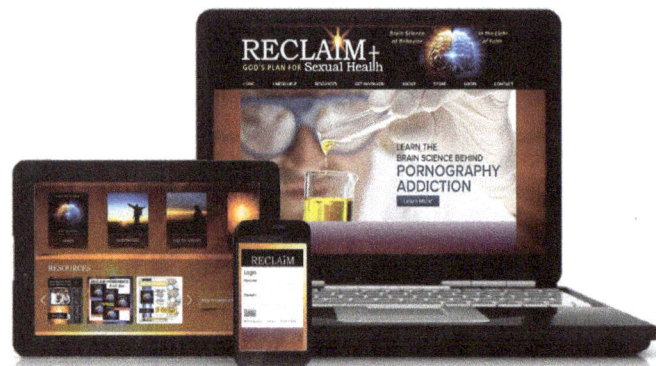

PLACE YOUR CHILD IN GOD'S HANDS

"Pray as if everything depends on God, work as if everything depends on you." (St. Ignatius of Loyola.)

Trust God and lift your child up to Him in prayer; then work tirelessly and urgently to do God's work in helping your child. Your child has been given free will by God, and nothing you do can take that away. Trusting the eventual outcome to God's loving care is the only way to find peace and security.

Note: *Due to limitation of space, we are not including many faith practices that may be helpful. Please seek out additional sources. Start with www.Catholic.org and www.usccb.org for information.*

DAILY PRACTICES

Avoiding unhealthy sexual behaviors will require a solid program of daily spiritual and practical exercises. Utilize the Scriptures, Sacraments, teachings of the saints, the Catechism of the Catholic Church, prayers, and sacramentals with a focus on the virtues, the Beatitudes, and the gifts of the Holy Spirit. These tools will teach your child self-mastery based on Catholic principles, and with God's grace, they will help him to apply that self-mastery in his life.

Morning Prayer: One way to begin a daily prayer routine is to pray with your child each morning. It can be as simple as:

"Good morning dear Jesus, today is for You. I ask You to bless all I think, say and do."

Add to this morning prayer time an Act of Consecration to the Immaculate Heart of Mary. *"O Virgin Mary, my Mother, I give to your Immaculate Heart my body and my soul, my thoughts and my actions. I want to be just what you want me to be, and do just what you want me to do. I am not afraid because you are always with me. Help me to love your Son, Jesus, with all my heart and above all things. Take my hand in yours, so I can always be with you."*

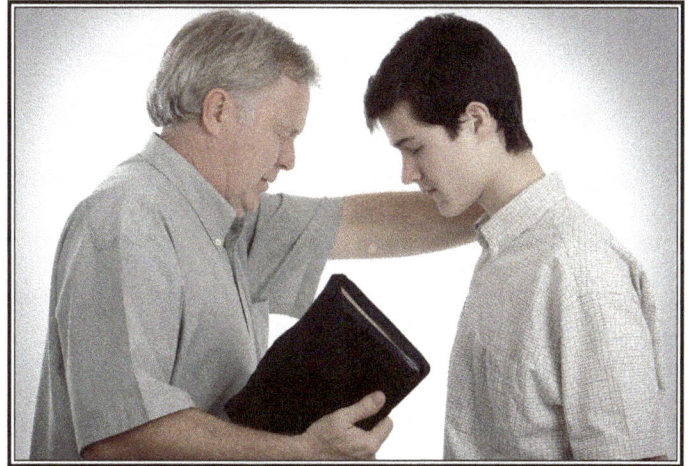

Blessing Prayer: Make it a daily practice to bless your child. This could be as simple as tracing the sign of the cross on your child's forehead, or placing your hands on him and saying a prayer such as: *"The light of God surrounds you; The love of God enfolds you; The power of God protects you; The presence of God watches over you; Where ever you are God is."* You can also pray a Scripture passage as a blessing:

"The LORD bless you and keep you!
The LORD let his face shine upon you, and be gracious to you! The LORD look upon you kindly and give you peace!"

Numbers 6:24-27

Meditative Prayer: Brain scientists have recently begun to study the effects of mediation on the brain. They have discovered meditation's ability to "retrain thought" can alter cognitive processing in the brain, produce natural stress-alleviation, and reduce the power of triggers and cravings in recovering individuals.[24] By incorporating the meditative and contemplative aspects of Catholic prayer, much healing may take place.

Dr. Mark Laaser, a well known expert on pornography addiction, shares a brain scan done on a pornography addict that showed considerable loss of function in the frontal cortex area of the brain. After a period of only twenty minutes of prayerful meditation of the rosary, blood flow was already beginning to return to that frontal area. This was confirmed by a second scan done immediately after the rosary was completed. *(Images of brains on next page provided by Dr. Mark Laaser.)[25]*

Healthy Brain **Addicted Brain**

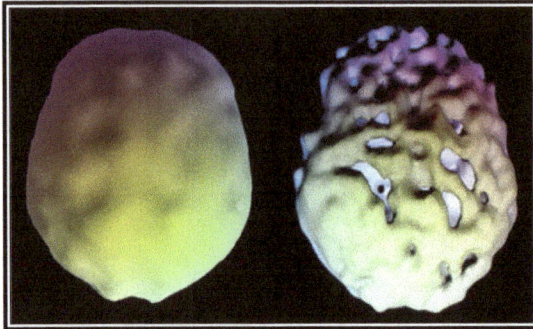

In Matthew 11: 28-30, Jesus gives a special invitation to all those who struggle, which most certainly includes those caught up in pornography or other unhealthy sexual behaviors.

"Come to me, all you who labor and are burdened, and I will give you rest. Take my yoke upon you and learn from me, for I am meek and humble of heart; and you will find rest for your selves. For my yoke is easy, and my burden light."

In this invitation, Jesus is also reaching out to you as a parent. You are not alone. Through your faith, and with God's divine help, you and your child will get through this and emerge more faith-filled.

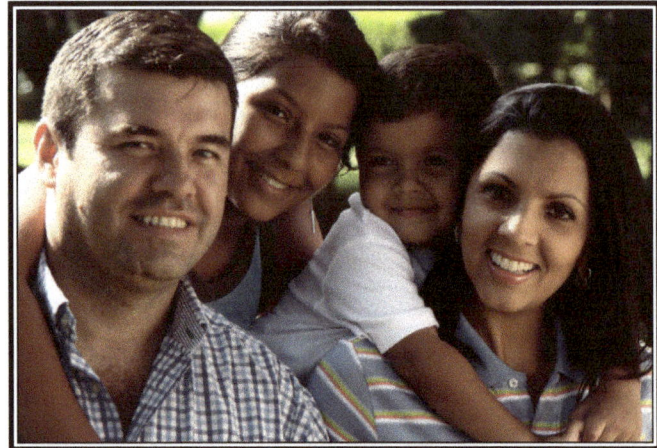

Keep in mind the words of Saint John Paul II;
*"We are not the sum of our failures,
but the sum of our Father's Love."*

RECLAIM GOD'S PLAN FOR SEXUAL HEALTH

WHAT IS GOD'S PLAN FOR SEXUALITY?

A 17-year-old woman in a high school class recently asked in all sincerity, "Wouldn't you die without sex?"

A 23-year-old college student travelled to Ireland with 20 classmates. She was one of only a few who didn't spend the evenings seeking hook-ups in pubs.

A woman decided that she is not female (even though she birthed children) but is rather a man – and with hormone therapy she now looks and sounds the part.

Confusion over sex is rampant today. Divergent opinions on and definitions of sexuality cause division in our nation, our churches, and even in our families. However, understanding sexuality is crucial to understanding God, ourselves and others. In fact, our take on sexuality impacts so much of our lives: how we live, our happiness, the future of humanity, and even our readiness for heaven.

SEX: ACCORDING TO THE CULTURE

Ask a friend to define the word "sexuality" or look up the word "sexuality" on the Internet and you will find a variety of complicated and confusing reactions. According to our culture sexuality is any and all of the following:

- the capacity for sexual feelings,

- a person's sexual orientation or preference,

- a tendency to be attracted to men, women, or both,

- a concern with or interest in sexual activity,

- the quality or state of being,

- a form of self-expression,

- a sense of masculinity or femininity that can change,

- an itch to be scratched.

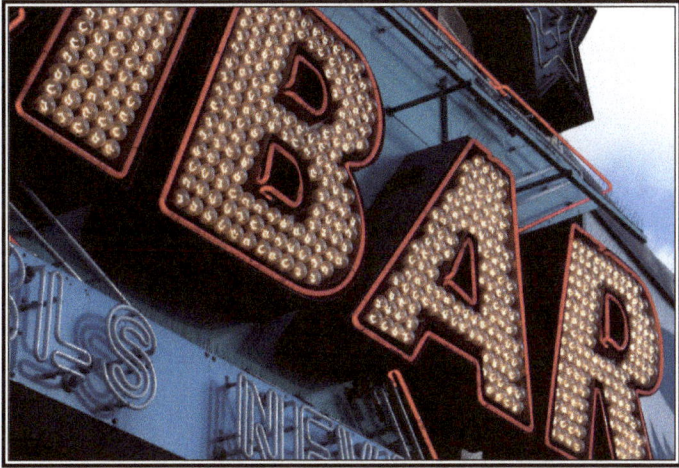

Current media's depiction of sex and sexuality doesn't help to clarify the matter. The TV, movie, and music industries incessantly depict sex as a powerful, almost irresistible force which draws people into intimacy with each other, and which enables them to experience passion and pleasure.

Despite the confusion that reigns when it comes to pinning down a single cultural definition of sexuality, there is a common thread: *My sexuality is all about me, and the goal of sex is for me to experience sexual release. Sexuality is such a driving and powerful force that sexual release is a necessity, and I have the right to experiencing that release however I want.*

This narcissistic (it's all about me), hedonistic (it's all about pleasure) and relativistic (no one is ever wrong) cultural attitude leads to a culture full of selfish, pleasure seeking, impulse driven individuals. This attitude is rooted in a diminished view of the human person and in a diminished view of human sexuality. You may recognize this cultural attitude toward sexuality in one of it's many mantras:

"You only live once."

"Avoid pain. Don't sacrifice."

"Hold on to what you've got."

"If it feels good, do it."

"What happens in my bedroom is my business."

The fruits of this attitude are heart wrenching: abortions, affairs, divorces, sexually transmitted infections, and wounded hearts, just to name a few. The breakdown of families and the absence of fathers caused by this attitude leads to wounded children who are more likely to struggle on all counts, especially later on in marriage. The refusal to sacrifice and to be generous in having children furthers the demographic winter in the western world where birth rates fall far below replacement rates. Economic stagnation and shrinkage result. Bigger governments develop to provide assistance that used to be provided by family members. Abortion and even euthanasia appear almost necessary as families and finances flounder. Clearly, these mantras and attitudes wander far away from the peace and joy found in recognizing who we are created to be, accepting our purpose in life, and living the true human vocation.

SEX ACCORDING TO GOD

To understand God's plan for sexuality we need to go back to the beginning – all the way to the story of creation in Genesis.

> Then God said: "Let us make man in our image, after our likeness. Let them have dominion over the fish of the sea, the birds of the air, and the cattle, and over all the wild animals and all the creatures that crawl on the ground." God created man in his image; in the divine image he created him; male and female he created them. God blessed them, saying: "Be fertile and multiply; fill the earth and subdue it. Have dominion over the fish of the sea, the birds of the air, and all the living things that move on the earth." (Genesis 1:26-28)

The story of our creation tells us about our purpose as beings created in the image and likeness of God. First, we learn that the God in whose image we were created is not just a "He" but a "We." Our God is a Trinity—a divine communion of love. The love between the three individual persons (Father, Son, and Holy Spirit) of this communion is so strong that it binds them as one being. The love from this divine communion is so powerful, that it creates life. We are created to be in relationships of divine communion with God and with others.

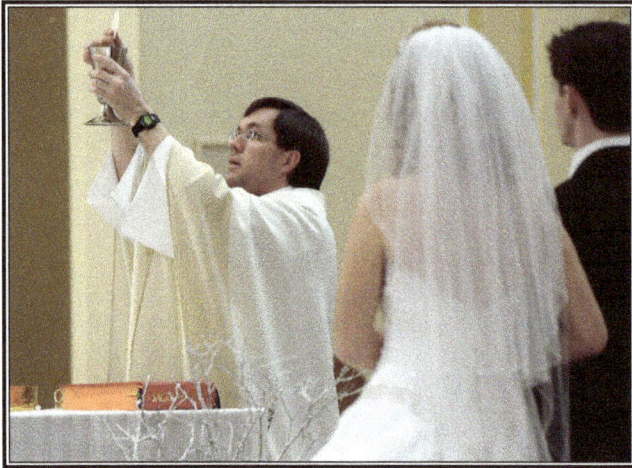

We also learn that we were created "male and female." The complementarity of the sexes is the physical sign that makes visible the invisible reality of our call to imitate and reflect the divine communion of the Trinity. The male and female bodies fit together in a way that makes them "one." All of creation mirrors His glory, but man and woman best illustrate who God is. His final creation is not an individual, but a unity between the two. Within the sacrament of marriage, the love of this divine communion is reflected so that the two male and female become one, and the love of this divine communion is imitated so that the relationship creates life.

Because we are created in the image of this beautiful and perfect communion of love, we long for love, we long for community, and we long for union. On the deepest level we long for union with our Creator – this is the eternal destiny to which we are invited. Our sexuality points us to heaven, which is union with God. However, God does not make us spend this entire life on earth waiting and hoping and longing. He gives us our sexuality as a means through which we can experience a taste of that union here on earth. He gives us a desire for human love and for physical intimacy—God gave us the desire for sex.

SEX: ACCORDING TO BIOLOGY

Our hunger, or longing, for human love is built into our bodies and minds. Our gender isn't incidental to who we are – it is essential. Every cell, even the smallest strand of DNA, reveals whether we are male or female. Men and women are different biologically, mentally and spiritually. They share the same human dignity, but they move through life and react to people and their environment in different ways. Each gender has a particular genius in the way it complements the other. Men are generally bigger and stronger; they are built to protect and provide; their thinking tends to be more linear and narrowly focused; and they tend to be problem solvers and task oriented. Women are built for nurturing; they are softer, more receptive; their thicker corpus callosum (which bridges the two hemispheres of the brain) enables them to efficiently multi-task; and they excel at taking care of relationships. These differences (and this just skims the surface) are both fascinating and significant.

The hedonistic, narcissistic and relativistic attitudes toward sex has often sought to minimize the differences between men and women in our culture. Radical feminists disdain and repress their femininity (especially their fertility, maternity, sensitivity, and receptivity), seeking instead strength and power. Men, whose masculinity has been slowly eroded by females who have undermined their natural strengths, end up confused. Women have told them to agree that a woman can do any job (even frontline warfare or the priesthood) that a man can do, but then are offended if he doesn't open the door for her.

This cultural attitude toward sexuality has lead many to completely disregard biology as insignificant. The physical realities and basic biological requirements of sexual union that have been written into our bodies by God are rejected as hedonistic desires take over. Whenever sexuality is turned away from the imitation and reflection of the life-creating love of the Trinity, the individual misses out on the purpose for which he or she was created.

The belief that we have a right to get what we want has led couples struggling with infertility, believing that they have a right to a child, to pursue in vitro fertilization, ignoring the centrality of the marital embrace. The physical union between a husband and a wife, renews the couple's commitment to their marriage vows and reminds them of the divine communion of love they are created for. When this loving act, which joins God and the couple, is removed from the creation of life, the couple no longer reflects and imitates divine communion of love for which they long.

God has written into our very biology the purpose for our sexuality. The purposes of sex are twofold and inseparable: the procreation of children (it reflects and imitates the life giving love of the Trinity) and the unity of the couple (it reflects and imitates the divine communion of the Trinity). Even when our culture tries to diminish or deny one of these purpose of sexuality, it cannot ignore biology. The culture wants to deny the procreative aspects of sex, promoting control of fertility. The biological fact is that it takes a man and a woman to conceive a child. The culture wants to diminish the unitive aspects of sex, substituting 'pleasure' for 'union.' The biological brain science of neurochemicals released during sex demonstrates that peaceful, fruitful union can only be experienced within the context of a marriage relationship.

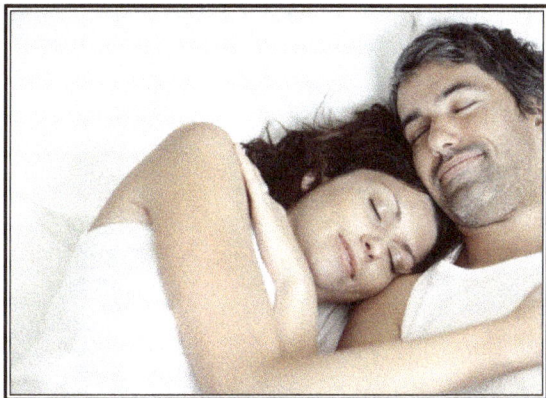

The biological realities illuminate deep truths about sex. Because the sexual embrace is the only natural way for procreation, and because the best outcomes for children are found in a home with their biological mother and father, the sexual embrace is to be reserved for marriage. Only in marriage do a man and woman commit to lifelong fidelity. Only in this lifelong commitment is it reasonable and prudent to give yourself entirely, totally, to your beloved. Only in this lifelong commitment is it appropriate to release the bonding neurochemicals experienced during sex. Cohabitating couples do not make this irrevocable commitment to each other.

A BETTER WAY

God's plan for our sexuality is a far cry from our pornographic hyper-sexualized culture which claims that everyone has a right to sex whenever they want it, that everyone has a right to either have or not have a baby by whatever means possible. Our culture suggests that freedom is to cater to those desires, to scratch when and where it itches. It proclaims that sex is a basic necessity, a right, an instinct which should usually be followed.

From our culture's perspective, God's plan for sexuality only within the context of sacramental marriage appears exclusive and limiting. If sex is a necessity and a right, then the call to freedom through self-mastery seems impossible and preposterous. If sex is all about selfish pleasure, then abstaining for any reason appears pointless. The fruits of this perspective are entrapment, anxiety and shame.

Consider the fruits of God's plan instead. God's plan for sexuality provides true freedom in that we are free to choose our actions rather than having them dictated to us by our sexual urges. God's plan works with the biology of our bodies instead of trying to subvert the natural order at every turn. It opens up the incredible and powerful gift of life and the possibility of becoming co-creators with God. God's plan provides for stable homes with mothers and fathers where children flourish. God's plan gives us a foretaste of the divine communion of love that we long for deep in our hearts.

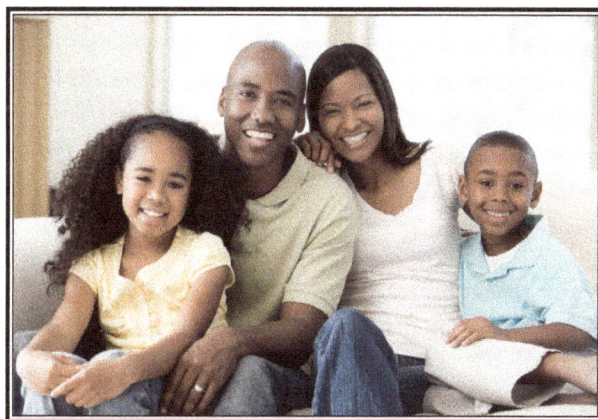

BETTER, BUT NOT ALWAYS EASY

Yes, there are parts that will be difficult, times when God's plan calls us to set aside our selfish desires in favor of sacrifice. God's plan calls all of us to chastity, to the successful integration of sexuality within ourselves. Whether married, single or consecrated to celibacy, following God's plan allows us to be in control of our urges and appetites rather than being a slave to them. The true freedom of God's plan is lived out according to our state of life. For the single, chastity will mean sexual abstinence until marriage. For the consecrated celibate, it will mean virginity for the sake of God's kingdom. For the married, chastity will keep the marital act always open to children (not using contraceptives) and always seeking union with the other (not using sex as a tool or a weapon). Sexual pleasure is morally disordered when sought for itself, isolated from its procreative and unitive purposes.

Chaste living is difficult at times for everyone, because hedonism (the desire to do whatever we feel like doing) has been so ingrained in us. However, the fruits of following God's plan for our sexuality instead of our culture's approach will be true joy, liberty, and holiness. Love and sexuality are topics that touch the core of every human heart. In today's society, understanding sexuality and what it means to love can be difficult. Scripture and the Church's teaching on these subjects are rich and full of good news.

For you were called for freedom, brothers. But do not use this freedom as an opportunity for the flesh; rather, serve one another through love. For the whole law is fulfilled in one statement, namely, "You shall love your neighbor as yourself." But if you go on biting and devouring one another, beware that you are not consumed by one another. I say, then: live by the Spirit and you will certainly not gratify the desire of the flesh. For the flesh has desires against the Spirit, and the Spirit against the flesh; these are opposed to each other, so that you may not do what you want. But if you are guided by the Spirit, you are not under the law. Now the works of the flesh are obvious: immorality, impurity, licentiousness, idolatry, sorcery, hatreds, rivalry, jealousy, outbursts of fury, acts of selfishness, dissensions, factions, occasions of envy, drinking bouts, orgies, and the like. I warn you, as I warned you before, that those who do such things will not inherit the kingdom of God. In contrast, the fruit of the Spirit is love, joy, peace, patience, kindness, generosity, faithfulness, gentleness, self-control. Against such there is no law. Now those who belong to Christ [Jesus] have crucified their flesh with its passions and desires. Galatians 5:13-24

In Benedict XVI's encyclical on love, he reminded us that the essence of love and life is found in Jesus' teaching that whoever loses his life will preserve it (Luke 17:33).[26] This may not sound like much fun – especially in the realm of sexuality, but this is precisely where it is the most important. In a speech to the Roman Curia in December, 2012, he said "Only in self-giving does man find himself, and only by opening himself to the other, to others, to children, to the family, only by letting himself be changed through suffering, does he discover the breadth of his humanity."[27]

We are sexual beings, created by Love, in the image of Love, for love, to love. Our sexuality doesn't just point the way to love; it is the way of love. Each man and woman is called to a life of noble, heroic, sacrificial love. Some will live out this calling in service to spouse and children, others to a parish or the community at large. Our sexuality is a gift from God. Once it is understood as a reflection of who God is and who we have been created to be in God's image, it becomes our gift back to God and to our neighbor. What impact will this teaching have on us and on our children? If we receive it, learn and live it – all the while relying on God's help – we will find that we are on the path to true freedom and abiding joy. This will go a long way not only in bringing us personal happiness, but will help rebuild marriage and family life, producing a culture of life and a civilization of love.

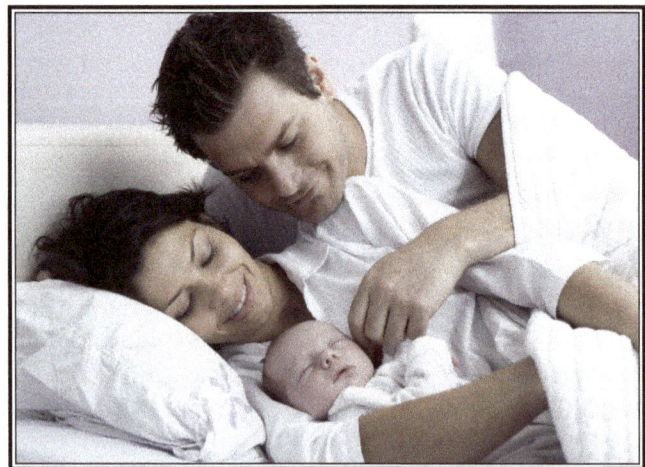

Note: Thank you for reading through this Parent Primer. We encourage you to get more information and help by visiting www.reclaimsexualhealth.com or calling us at 920.766.9380.

NOTES

1. *The Brain That Changes Itself,* Dr. Norman Doidge, Viking Penguin, 2007.

2. *"Social Media & Mobile Internet Use among Teens and Adults,"* Pew Internet and American Life Project, 2007, hhtp://www.pewinternet.org.

3. *The Drug of the New Millennium-Brain Science Behind Internet Pornography Use,* Mark Kastleman, Power Think Publishing, 2007.

4. *"Social Media & Mobile Internet,"* Amanda Lenhart, Pew Internet and American Life Project, 2007, http://www.pwerinternet.org.

5. *Hearing on Pornography's Impact on Marriage & The Family,* Dr. Jill C. Manning, Testimony, Subcommittee on the Constitution, Civil Rights, and Property Rights, Committee on Judiciary, United States Senate. Nov. 10, 2005

6. *Porn-Induced Sexual Dysfunction: A Growing Problem,* Marnia Robinson, Psychology Today, July 11, 2011, http://www.psychologytoday.com.

7. Senate Testimony 2004 by Jill Manning, referencing: Dedmon, J., "Is the Internet bad for your marriage? Online affairs, pornographic sites playing greater role in divorces," 2002, press release from the Dilenschneider Group, Inc.

8. *"The Pornography Pandemic,"* Patrick Trueman, Knights of Columbus Columbia Magazine, 10/28/2011, http://www.kofc.org/en/columbia/detail/2011_11_computer.html

9. *"Pornography Statistics,"* Covenant Eyes Accountability and Filtering, 2013, http://www.covenanteyes.com/pornstats/

10. Internet Filter Review, 2004

11. Conversation with a mother and Jeannie Hannemann. To learn more about this game, go to: Public Broadcasting Service, http://natbott97.wordpress.com/2013/03/07/pbs-idea-channel-is-minecraft-the-ultimate-educational-tool/

12. Clinical work of Dr. Mark Chamberlain, http://markchamberlainphd.blogspot.com

13. *The Drug of the New Millennium-Brain Science Behind Internet Pornography Use,* Mark Kastleman, Power Think Publishing, 2007. (The BLHASTED acronym was created by therapist Dan Gray.

14. JAMA and Archives Journals. *"Psychiatric Symptoms May Predict Internet Addiction In Adolescents."* ScienceDaily. 6 October 2009. <www.sciencedaily.com/releases/2009/10/091005181636.htm>.

15. http://www.drjudithreisman.com/erototoxin.html

16. *Parenting with Grace: Catholic Parent's Guide to Raising Almost Perfect Kids,* Gregory K. Popcak and Lisa Popcak, Our Sunday Visitor, 2010

17. Satinover, J. (2004). Senate Committee on Commerce, Science, and Transportation, Subcommittee on Science, Technology, and Space, *Hearing on the Brain Science Behind Pornography Addiction and Effects of Addiction on Families and Communities,* November 18.

18. Yuan, K., Quin, W., Lui, Y., and Tian, J. (2011). *Internet Addiction: Neuroimaging Findings.* Communicative & Integrative Biology 4, 6: 637–639; Zhou, Y., Lin, F., Du, Y., Qin, L., Zhao, Z., Xu, J., et al. (2011). *Gray Matter Abnormalities in Internet Addiction: A Voxel-Based Morphometry Study.* European Journal of Radiology 79, 1: 92–95; Miner, M. H., Raymond, N., Mueller, B. A., Lloyd, M., Lim, K. O. (2009). *Preliminary Investigation of the Impulsive and Neuroanatomical Characteristics of Compulsive Sexual Behavior.* Psychiatry Research 174: 146–51; Schiffer, B., Peschel, T., Paul, T., Gizewshi, E., Forshing, M., Leygraf, N., et al. (2007). *Structural Brain Abnormalities in the Frontostriatal System and Cerebellum in Pedophilia.* Journal of Psychiatric Research 41, 9: 754–762; Pannacciulli, N., Del Parigi, A., Chen, K., Le, D. S. N. T., Reiman, R. M., and Tataranni, P. A. (2006). *Brain Abnormalities in Human Obesity: A Voxel-Based Morphometry Study.* NeuroImage 31, 4: 1419–1425.

19. Doidge, N. (2007). *The Brain That Changes Itself.* New York: Penguin Books, 107.

20. Hilton, D. L. (2013). *Pornography Addiction—A Supranormal Stimulus Considered in the Context of Neuroplasticity.* Socioaffective Neuroscience & Psychology 3:20767; Pfaus, J. (2011). *Love and the Opportunistic Brain.* In The Origins of Orientation, World Science Festival, June. Georgiadis, J. R. (2006). *Regional Cerebral Blood Flow Changes Associated with Clitorally Induced Orgasm in Healthy Women.* European Journal of Neuroscience 24, 11: 3305–3316.

21. Paul, P. (2007). *Pornified: How Pornography Is Transforming Our Lives, Our Relationships, and Our Families.* New York: Henry Hold and Co., 90.

22. Wallace, D. L., Vialou, V., Rios, L., Carle-Florence, T. L., Chakravarty, S., Kumar, A., et al. (2008). *The Influence of DeltaFosB in the Nucleus Accumbens on Natural Reward-Related Behavior.* The Journal of Neuroscience 28: 10272–7; Nestler, E. J. (2003). *Brain Plasticity and Drug Addiction.* Presentation at Reprogramming the Human Brain Conference, Center for Brain Health, University of Texas at Dallas, April 11.

23. Sturman, D. and Moghaddam, B. (2011). *Reduced Neuronal Inhibition and Coordination of Adolescent Prefrontal Cortex during Motivated Behavior.* The Journal of Neuroscience 31, 4: 1471-1478.)

24. *Meditation's Role In Drug Addiction Recovery,* June 9, 2011, http://www.neurosoup.com/meditation_and_addiction.htmStudy cited from US National Library of Medicine—National Institutes of Health, http://www.ncbi.nlm.nih.gov/pubmed/16938074

25. *Faithful and True Ministry,* Dr. Mark Laaser, PhD, http://www.faithful and true.com

26. God Is Love, Deus Caritas Est, Encyclical Letter, Pope Benedict XVI, 2006, USCCB Publication No. 5-758.

27. Address of His Holiness Benedict XVI Christmas Greeting to the Roman Curia, Friday, 21 December 2012, http://www.vatican.va/holy_father/benedict_xvi/speeches/2012/december/documents/hf_ben-xvi_spe_20121221_auguri-curia_en.html

Letter to Families, Pope John Paul II http://www.vatican.va/holy_father/john_paul_ii/letters/documents/hf_jp-ii_let_02021994_families_en.html

Scripture quotes taken from *New American Bible.*
Used with permission.

ABOUT THE PARENT PRIMER RECLAIM TEAM AUTHORS

Kristin Bird, M.A.
Kristin Bird, M.A. has worked for many years in multiple parish settings as a youth minister and High School Ministry Coordinator. She is a skilled presenter and serves as a consultant to many faith based organizations. Kristin graduated with degrees in English, Spanish, Religious Studies and Secondary Education. She has a Master's Degree in Pastoral Studies. Kristin serves as an *Elizabeth Ministry* Consultant.

Bruce Hannemann, M.A.
As an author and public speaker, Bruce has shared his own pornography recovery story with humility and candor. He is honored to tell his experience of God's restoration in his life and marriage. Bruce brings a wealth of understanding of young adults and the ability to teach scientific concepts with over thirty years experience teaching science at the college level. Bruce earned a Master's Degree in *Adult Christian Community Development* with a concentration on *Adult Learning.* His understanding of *Theology of the Body* combined with training in sex addiction recovery, brain science and the biochemistry of sexuality has put an end to the mystery of lust and given him a way to share how to reclaim God's plan for sexuality with proven answers that have touched the lives of many. His witty personality, genuine compassion and ability to take complex topics and teach them in a down to earth manner has made him a popular presenter.

Jeannie Hannemann, M.A.
Jeannie has over thirty-five years experience assisting families through a variety of formats, including as an educator, parish pastoral and family life minister, Catholic radio talk show host, consultant and retreat director. Jeannie has a Master's Degree in *Adult Christian Community Development* with a concentration in *Family Life.* Jeannie's personal journey through her husband's pornography addiction, training in sexual addiction recovery, extensive family life ministry experiences, and her belief in the power of God's grace makes her a sought after confidant and presenter. As the founder of Elizabeth Ministry, she is an internationally recognized author and speaker. Her programs have won diocesan, and national awards within the church and secular community. Drawing from lived experiences, advanced training and faith, she offers practical tools to help people make wise life decisions, emotional tools for developing healthy relationships and spiritual tools to transform pain to peace.

Mark Kastleman
Mark Kastleman has conducted training for professionals across the U.S. and in various parts of the world. His audiences have included top government officials, psychologists, therapists, medical doctors, educators, law enforcement and the military. Mark is recognized for his writing in the areas of brain science and behavioral change, following in the footsteps of his mentor, world-renowned neuropsychologist, Dr. Page Bailey. Mark has received international acclaim for his extensive work in the field of pornography addiction prevention and recovery. His book *The Drug of the New Millennium, The Brain Science Behind Internet Pornography Use* is widely cited and utilized by therapists, counselors and clergy. In addition to his professional background, Mark brings a unique perspective and experience to his role on the RECLAiM team through his own 25-year struggle and successful recovery from sexual addiction.

Carol Quist, M.Th. and Paul Quist, MDiv, STL
Paul Quist (former Lutheran pastor) and his wife Carol enthusiastically spread the good news about marriage, family, sexuality and the human person which they discovered in the Catholic Church. At mid-life, they moved their family to Melbourne, Australia to study at the John Paul II Institute for Marriage and Family. Carol earned a Master of Theology in Marriage and Family and Paul completed his studies with a sacred theology licence (STL) from the Lateran Pontifical University in Rome. Paul was director of the Office of Marriage and Family Life for the Archdiocese of Edmonton. Now he and Carol lead marriage and family ministries at Holy Trinity Catholic Church in Spruce Grove, Alberta, and Paul teaches part-time at Newman Theological College in Edmonton. They have three children in their early twenties and late teens.

Chris Sperling, M.A. L.M.F.T.
Chris is a Licensed Marriage & Family Therapist in the state of Texas. As a trained sexual addiction therapist, he provides treatment to individuals, couples & families who are struggling with negative sexual behaviors that effect the relational, occupational and/or legal spheres of their lives. Chris is also a trained EMDR therapist and uses this brain based protocol to work with clients who struggle with problematic sexual behavior. Chris is part of the RECLAiM Professional Team and successfully implements the RECLAiM recovery process in his therapy.

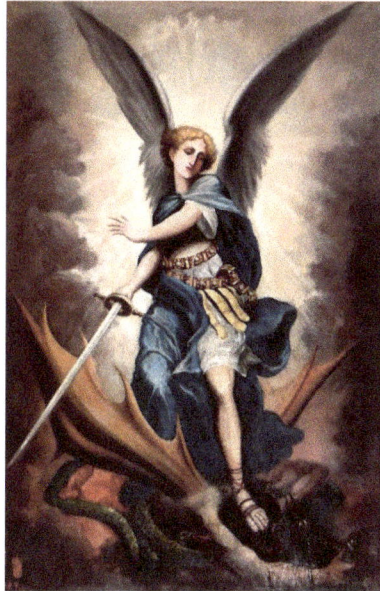

St. Michael Prayer

Saint Michael the Archangel,
defend us in battle.
Be our protection against
the wickedness and snares of the devil.
May God rebuke him, we humbly pray;
and do Thou, O Prince of the Heavenly Host,
by the Divine Power of God,
cast into hell Satan and all the evil spirits
who roam throughout the world
seeking the ruin of souls.
Amen.